THE
TERRENCE HIGGINS TRUST
HIV/AIDS BOOK

JUDY TAVANYAR

Thorsons
An Imprint of HarperCollins*Publishers*

Thorsons
An Imprint of HarperCollins*Publishers*
77-85 Fulham Palace Road,
Hammersmith, London W6 8JB

Published by Thorsons 1992
1 3 5 7 9 10 8 6 4 2

A catalogue record for this book
is available from the British Library

ISBN 0 7225 2540 0

Typeset by Harper Phototypesetters Limited,
Northampton, England
Printed in Great Britain by
Mackays of Chatham, Kent

CONTENTS

ACKNOWLEDGEMENTS

I would like to acknowledge the help, advice and information given by a wide range of individuals and organisations with the preparation of this book. Space does not allow me to give the names of everybody who has been involved, but I would like to include the following:

Tina Bird, Liz Dibb, Robin Dormer, Heather Downs, Andrea Efthimiou, Janet Green, Richard Haigh, Lauren Jackson, Ben Kernighan, Judy Mariasy, Gavin McKivragan, Colin Nee, Nick Partridge, Marty Radlett, Simmy Viniika, Jim Wilson, and staff in the Terrence Higgins Trust library who kept me supplied with press cuttings and other materials.

Special thanks go to Ruth Parry, who read and made comments on early drafts of this book, to Corinne Pearlman for her illustrations, to Caroline Akehurst for her generous supply of information, and to Clare Gilpin for her unfailing support, encouragement and love.

By publisher's request, this book is not referenced. Some of the literature that has been most useful in its preparation is listed at the back. However, some publications deserve special mention here. *The National AIDS Manual* ~ Peter Scott et al., *The AIDS Handbook* ~ Carl Miller, *The Search for the Virus* ~ Steve Connor and Sharon Kingman, *Information File* ~ National AIDS Prevention and Information Service, *Safer Sex* ~ Peter Gordon and Louise Mitchell, *Living with AIDS and HIV* ~ David Miller, *Caring for Someone with AIDS* ~ Research Institute for Consumer Affairs/Disabilities Study Unit, *The Third Epidemic* and *Triple Jeopardy* ~ Panos Institute. I have drawn information in particular from *The AIDS Newsletter* published by the AIDS Unit at the Bureau of Hygiene and Tropical Diseases, as from the Terrence Higgins Trust's *HIV News Review* throughout the preparation of this book, and (for Chapter 9) from *World AIDS*, a bi-monthly magazine published by the Panos Institute.

An extra special thank-you has to go to Abby Daniels, the Drugs Training Officer at the Terrence Higgins Trust, who did an outstanding job of proof-reading and contributing towards the completion of the book.

INTRODUCTION

The Terrence Higgins Trust (THT) was set up in 1983 in memory of Terrence Higgins, one of the first people to die with AIDS in the UK. Its purpose was to provide support, information and advice to those people affected, directly and indirectly, by HIV and AIDS. As the number of people affected by this virus has increased, THT has grown in order to accommodate their needs. THT started as a helpline service. In addition it now provides legal, housing and Welfare Benefit advice and advocacy, buddying, practical help with such things as decorating, cleaning and transportation, counselling, support for HIV-positive prisoners and drug users, health education and information.

The HIV epidemic has raised questions about so many aspects of the way we live our lives. Attitudes to sex and sexuality, drug taking, illness, death and bereavement – subjects that for many of us may be shrouded in embarrassment, ignorance and fear – have come under its harsh spotlight. Ten years after the term 'AIDS' was first coined by doctors in the US, there are still no easy answers to some of these questions. However, an enormous amount of knowledge and insight has been gained, and considerable advances in both preventing and treating HIV infection have been made.

In the search for help and information about the questions and issues raised by HIV, thousands of people have contacted the Terrence Higgins Trust in the nine years since it was set up. I have assumed that you, the reader, could be any one of the people who has done so or who may wish to do so in the future. The range of this book is therefore as broad as possible. If you have concerns and questions about any aspect of HIV or AIDS and would also like to know how to get further guidance and advice, then this book is written for you.

For those people who are not infected with HIV, behavioural change is the only protection available against the virus. Until there is a vaccine or a safe and efficient drug to control the impact of HIV on the body, education about safer behaviour is the strongest medicine we can offer. Yet education does not take place in a vacuum. We cannot ignore the personal factors that affect an individual's behaviour; sexual autonomy within relationships, social and economic status, cultural and religious beliefs.

Such questions are impossible to address adequately in a book of this sort. What it does propose to do is dispense with some of the myths that have dogged our ability to reflect upon HIV without a sense of hopelessness and panic, and thus perhaps represent a starting-point for further exploration. It might also raise some important questions about our understanding of health and social responsibility, by focussing on the possibilities offered by fuller information on relevant issues. Must we, for example, understand appropriate health care to be the territory of 'experts', or can patients get involved, make choices, demand to know more?

As has been written elsewhere, public perceptions of HIV have been shaped by the metaphors that surround it. A simple package of cells in a membrane envelope has been widely and dangerously over-interpreted by people with a moral (and sometimes racial) axe to grind. Thus, HIV infection has been presented to us as God's punishment to the 'unworthy' (such as gay men and drug users), or the well-deserved price of what some see as the sexual licentiousness of the 'permissive sixties'; a kind of come-uppance for those judged to have spent too much time enjoying themselves by those who may not have enjoyed themselves enough. As Lord Kilmarnock, chair of the All-Party Parliamentary Group on AIDS, has stated, 'We put more faith in condoms than sermons.'

The reality is that HIV cannot select 'targets', choose 'victims', or map out a course of destruction against our will in the way that we may have sometimes been led to believe. This book is about staying healthy; it is about living well, whether we are HIV negative or positive. We do not have to let a distorting screen of inappropriate images make us passive and powerless in the face of this epidemic.

The last word in this introduction goes to John Mordaunt, who has lived with an AIDS diagnosis for several years. To him, as to all people with HIV, this book is dedicated.

The best surprise for me was when I realised I was OK. I have a viral illness, that's all. I don't have a moral illness, I don't have a deficiency of the soul. I'm a true human being who is dealing with a difficult situation in the best way he can.

January 1992

1

FROM IGNORANCE TO HOPE

THE STORY OF HIV IN BRITAIN

I know that many people at first refused to believe that a crisis was
upon us. I know, because I was one of them.
*– Halfdan Mahler, former Director General of
the World Health Organization*

WHAT'S IN A NAME?

The story of HIV and AIDS is one of scientific brilliance and
linguistic obscurity. Since the condition which we now call AIDS
was first discovered in the United States in 1981, the expertise and
energy put into studying its causes and progression have been
unprecedented in the history of medicine. There is now optimistic
discussion of developing a vaccine by the end of this century which
will prevent infection with HIV and delay the development of
disease in people already infected with the virus. As research
continues into anti-viral treatments and drugs to control the effects
of related illnesses, it becomes increasingly likely that infection with
the human immunodeficiency virus (HIV) will become a chronic
but treatable condition rather than a life-threatening and incurable
one.

Such laudable advances make it easy to forget the uncertainty and
confusion of the early years of the epidemic. When US doctors first
came across patients with strange illnesses that are rarely seen in
healthy people, they knew nothing about the condition they were
examining or what could have caused it. The first scientific paper
on the subject highlighted the presence of an extremely rare type
of pneumonia in young men from Los Angeles caused by infection
of the lungs with a microorganism called *pneumocystis carinii*. Later
reports mentioned the discovery of a rare type of skin cancer called
Kaposi's sarcoma in 26 men from the west and east coasts of the
United States. The patients in each case had several things in

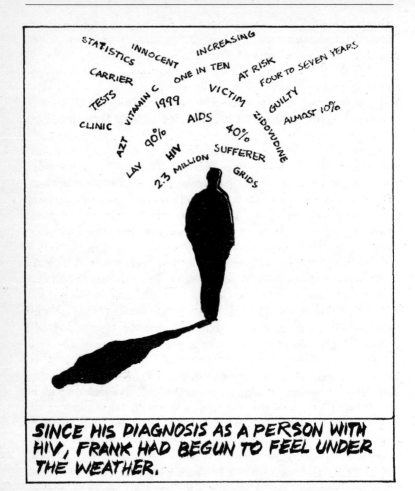

SINCE HIS DIAGNOSIS AS A PERSON WITH HIV, FRANK HAD BEGUN TO FEEL UNDER THE WEATHER.

common: they were young, male, appeared to be suffering from a weakened immune system, and mainly identified as being gay.

In the absence of any further concrete information, doctors decided to give the puzzling and apparently incurable new condition a name. This, as it turned out, would be their first mistake. They called it GRIDS: gay-related immune deficiency syndrome.

It is possible to understand the compulsion behind the GRIDS label: naming a mystifying phenomenon can confer a feeling of increased understanding, the exercise of some degree of control. Yet, even when the name was created, there was evidence from other scientific papers that the symptoms and infections related to GRIDS had been noted in people other than gay men.

By the time GRIDS was changed to AIDS (Acquired Immune Deficiency Syndrome) in 1982, significant damage had been done to public understanding and attitudes to people affected by the virus. The GRIDS label had established for those who wished to believe it that only gay men were at risk; they were, after all, the first people reported to be affected by AIDS in the US (and later in parts of Western Europe). It began a kind of tribal interpretation of the epidemic whereby infection risks and (by extension) responsibility for the spread of the virus came to be viewed as the property of specific social groups. The fact that the condition was noted in gay men, injecting drug users, people with haemophilia who had received contaminated blood products for treatment and people from Haiti led to early jokes about the four Hs as standard 'targets' for the virus (heroin users, homosexuals, haemophiliacs and Haitians), which caused an international row.

When it became clear over the following years that sexual and social identity (as opposed to behaviour) were irrelevant as far as HIV and AIDS are concerned, those who had at first refused to believe that they could be at risk began to look for a scapegoat when they realised they were wrong. Ten years on, the notion of 'risk groups' for HIV prevails.

Even the AIDS acronym has enforced misconceptions about the nature of HIV infection. The definition of AIDS established by doctors has tended to be seen as the 'final stage' of HIV disease and does not recognise that it is quite possible to die from HIV-related illness without having the specific symptoms that fit an AIDS diagnosis. Unfortunately, statistical reports tend to present the scale of the epidemic in terms of reported AIDS cases and deaths. (The number of people with HIV infection on a national or global basis, the majority of whom may be quite healthy, is at best an educated guess.) The distinction between HIV infection and AIDS is explored in more detail in Chapter 2, but it is quite possible that in the future the term AIDS may be discarded altogether, as its usefulness is increasingly questionable.

Naming HIV, the virus that can cause AIDS, also resulted in confusion and dissent. The virus was not identified until 1983 and no universally acceptable name found for it until 1986. By that stage, it became necessary to involve an international committee of researchers to make an agreement about what the virus should be called, since there were already at least two other terms for it in use. A team of US scientists led by Dr Robert Gallo, the head of a laboratory at the National Cancer Institute in Bethesda, Maryland, called the virus human T-cell lymphotropic virus type 3, or HTLV3, because it appeared to affect T lymphocyte cells in the blood of humans.

At the same time, French scientists led by Dr Luc Montagnier at the Pasteur Institute referred to the virus as lymphadenopathy AIDS-associated virus, or LAV. The acceptance of an internationally appropriate label was one outcome of a longstanding and bitter argument between Gallo and Montagnier, both of whom claimed to have been first to isolate and identify the virus which can cause AIDS. A legal settlement was reached in 1987 which presented Gallo and Montagnier as co-discoverers of what we now refer to as HIV.

BEGINNINGS

The first person with AIDS in the UK was reported in 1981. Five years of silence followed. It was not until March 1986 that the Government launched its first nation-wide campaign to educate the public about the risks of HIV infection. Newspaper advertisements told the public 'Don't Aid AIDS', but gave little clear information about how this could be done. The low-budget campaign resulted in uninspired advertisements, using euphemistic language. Market research suggested that some readers were left more confused about AIDS than they had been before the ads came out. It was thus hard to ignore the stark irony of one of the slogans of the Government's first campaign – 'AIDS: How Big Does it Have to Get before You Take Notice?'

So why had the British Government waited five years before bringing AIDS and HIV to the attention of the public? The answer can hardly lie in statistics alone. Even though the number of people with AIDS seemed relatively small by the end of 1986 – 610 cases in total – ministers had only to look at the American experience of the epidemic, where cases reached over 28,000 by the end of 1986, to realise what might lie ahead.

It is also hard to believe that the Government was ignorant of the likely future cost of care for people with HIV. Economists had already done their sums. Initial estimates from Department of Health (DoH) officials that it would cost about £10,000 a year to treat one person with AIDS had to be revised upwards to £20,000 a year in 1988, or £25,000 if new drug therapies were taken into account. The Office of Health Economics calculated in 1986 that treating people with AIDS in the UK would present the

Government with a bill of between £20 million and £30 million by 1988. (The actual cost to date for the period 1986–1991 has been £373 million for health care alone; this does not include the further £300 million spent on research, social services, etc.). Furthermore, these figures did not even begin to include the cost of work days lost due to HIV-related illnesses.

The global cost of the virus in terms of human misery – the impact of discrimination and prejudice, disruption of families and communities, illness, death and bereavement – was (and still is) immeasurable. As the rising toll of AIDS cases reported monthly by the World Health Organization (WHO) indicated, the problems posed by the epidemic were not going to disappear.

Perhaps the potential scale of the problem was so enormous that it had a paralysing effect upon ministers' sensibilities. However, the key to Government inaction is more likely to lie in the demographic impact of HIV. Had politicians felt that the epidemic was an issue of concern to those they regarded as making up the majority of the general electorate (in other words, heterosexual men and women), they may well have wished to take a determined stand earlier on. As it was, the vast majority of people dying with AIDS in the UK in the early years were gay men and (particularly in Scotland) injecting drug users, groups often viewed as somehow 'outside' the general population. MPs were well aware that it might not help their image to show too much concern for the needs of such marginalised communities.

By the mid-1980s the Government must have finally realised that the National Health Service could not afford what could easily become a devastating epidemic. The absence of clear, unsensational-ised information had, however, already taken its toll. Dangerous misunderstandings had developed about HIV transmission risks, so that where some felt that casual social contact – such as shaking hands, or having a drink – with a person with HIV could put them at risk, others assumed that the virus could have no impact upon their lives, whatever their sexual or drug-using behaviour. Easy phrases such as 'high-risk group', 'reservoir of infection' and 'heterosexual explosion' dominated discussion of AIDS, so that the public's vision of the epidemic was built upon the ideas of division and recrimination.

Ironically, those who had taken responsibility since 1982 for offering support, advice, information and counselling for anyone concerned about HIV and AIDS would not themselves be the focus of a DoH education campaign until 1989. For the first few years of the HIV epidemic, services organised by the gay community (many of whom were forced to stand by and watch as friends, lovers and family members died) were run without Government funding of any sort. While politicians recognised that education about HIV might be a considerably cheaper option than a mounting bill for hospital and community care, drug treatments and social services for people with HIV, they cannot have failed to notice how very cheap the education and support services provided by gay men and lesbians had already been.

BREAKING THE SILENCE

The first AIDS service organisation to be set up in the UK was named after Terry Higgins, a gay man who died in London in 1982, a long time before many people had any idea that the condition existed. Higgins' lover and friends, tired of the ignorance and prejudice that surrounded AIDS and the lack of services that his death had highlighted, decided to form the Terrence Higgins Trust (THT) to provide information and help to other people directly affected by or worried about AIDS.

Organising relevant services in such a situation was a major exercise in working with uncertainty. Workers at THT knew from what was happening in the US that the increasing number of AIDS cases reported each month was only the beginning, that what could follow was largely unquantifiable. Fund-raising for HIV education and support took the form of bucket-rattling and benefit evenings in gay bars and clubs; the first attempts to plan counselling and information work were conducted from people's houses, overcrowded offices and rooms above pubs - whatever space happened to be available.

While money and premises were hard to come by, so was reliable information. The way to avoid developing AIDS was largely open to guesswork. Those undertaking information and advice work at organisations like THT and (as it was then called) the London Gay Switchboard were confronted with a situation where they had to handle other people's anxieties and confusion about the strange new condition as well as coping with their own fears and the inevitable questions that lurked behind them. Could a disease really only affect people of the same sexuality? Did this mean that gay men should stop having sex altogether? If numbers of people with AIDS were still relatively low, would it perhaps be better to play the condition down?

By 1984, Gay Switchboard had organised the UK's first seminar on AIDS and the Gay Medical Association had produced the first leaflet on the issue. The first television programme to look at the subject, *Killer in the Village* by the BBC's *Horizon* team, revealed the effect AIDS was having on the gay community in New York City's Greenwich Village. A growing sense of purpose and collaboration was evident between volunteers and professionals involved in AIDS work. THT, which by now had its own offices and a formal charitable status, held its first annual conference in late 1984. The event established links and cemented relationships which would hold good for the years ahead. People with AIDS spoke about their experiences; doctors met gay activists and workers from the fields of haemophilia and drug use. The beginnings of an informal network of voluntary bodies came into being - groups in cities as far apart as Brighton and Edinburgh were taking action on AIDS.

In 1985, an organisation called *Body Positive* was set up by HIV-positive men and women to share the support and counselling work offered by the THT. It was followed a year later by *Frontliners*, a campaigning, information and support organisation which ran services by and for people with AIDS. People with HIV were tired of hearing themselves described as 'victims', 'sufferers' and 'carriers', and of seeing themselves represented in the media as emaciated figures on the brink of death. They wanted to challenge the negative images that bear no resemblance to the way many HIV-positive people feel and look, and do nothing to quieten the panic and hostility of others. Those who have direct experience of living and dealing with the virus are in a strong position to challenge public misconceptions. The work of people with HIV in the fields of advocacy and education since the early 1980s has brought about significant changes; it may have had far more impact upon public awareness and behaviour change than the most expensive media advertisements.

DISEASE AS PUNISHMENT

Although the arrival of AIDS had not *created* an atmosphere of hostility and prejudice towards gay men and lesbians (that was already there), it had certainly provided bigots and moralists with material to back their beliefs. Reporting of AIDS was taking on a disquietingly interpretative stance, suggesting that it was somehow much more than a medical condition. As the epidemic progressed and it became evident that the virus which could cause AIDS was transmitted through blood as well as sexual fluids, the notion of disease as punishment became clearly defined. Children infected by their mothers, people who became HIV positive through contaminated blood and blood products – these were deemed to be 'innocent victims' of the virus. The flip side of that theory was that gay men, drug users, and the 'sexually promiscuous' were, in some sense, 'guilty'. According to such representations, people with a life-threatening infection could appropriately be divided into two moral camps, one of which merited medical attention and support while the other did not.

In 1985, AIDS hit the headlines with force. Grim photographs and copy illustrating Rock Hudson's diagnosis shocked people who had chosen to see the condition as the exclusive property of a social underclass. It took the illness of a film-star to bring home the reality that AIDS was no respecter of wealth, privilege or success. In fact, from the tone of much of the tabloid coverage, it was clear that Hudson was affected by not one, but two conditions: AIDS and the stigma and humiliation with which, for journalists and many others, it was associated.

Shame and sickness were easy subjects for sensationalism. From the mid- to late 1980s, speculative stories about mythical HIV transmission routes appeared regularly; it was often possible to read totally contradictory accounts of what was and was not safe in terms of HIV infection from different papers on the same day.

It was as though AIDS, by challenging medical knowledge, was also challenging medical credibility. If doctors could not come up with a cure for the condition, if they did not really know how the virus made people ill – then could anything they said be trusted? People who regarded modern medicine as the domain of 'experts', doctors who would provide their clients with the security of an existence sealed off from pain and disease, had suffered a rude awakening in the age of AIDS.

TESTING TIMES

By 1985 it was at last becoming possible to take a test to find out whether or not you had been exposed to HIV infection. The test kits, which measured the presence of antibodies to HIV rather than the virus itself, were made available for screening blood donations in the UK almost six months after a similar test had been developed in the US. Minister of Health Kenneth Clarke excused the delay by saying that there were doubts over the reliability of American tests, which tended to produce a high number of 'false positive' results (in other words, they detected antibodies to HIV infection where none were present).

Many people regarded the decision to wait before introducing blood screening in the UK as untenable, on the grounds that it was better to have a test kit that allowed a few extra false positives than no method whatsoever for protecting the nation's blood supply from infected donations. Furthermore, anxious people who wished to take the HIV antibody test to find out whether they had the virus or not had suffered what could be seen as an unnecessary wait. In effect, the delay had given the British pharmaceuticals company Wellcome a chance to develop its own diagnostic test. This opened up a market estimated to be worth up to £200 million world-wide by the late 1980s, one previously dominated by American companies.

Even when HIV antibody testing was made available on a voluntary basis to individuals, AIDS workers knew it was not going to provide any easy solutions to slowing the spread of the epidemic. It was never going to be possible to 'test' HIV out of existence and, in any case, now the key transmission routes of the virus had been established, education materials could help people to practise safer behaviour whether they knew their HIV antibody status or not.

AIDS AND THE MEDIA

By late 1986, the Government could see that it would need to develop an AIDS strategy for the years ahead. A special Cabinet Committee was set up, the first of its kind to deal with a specific disease. The trouble was, so many factors that would determine the scale of the epidemic could not be calculated. Would people switch to safer sex and drug use to protect themselves? Would scientists be able to find a vaccine or an effective treatment for infection in the next five to ten years? If records were only kept of the number of people with AIDS, how many more were HIV positive but had not yet become ill? It is not surprising that when the Government launched its second public education campaign in 1987, this time involving television as well as press, billboards and a national leaflet mailing, one of the key images to appear in the advertisements was the tip of an enormous iceberg.

In many ways the 1987 campaign, which used the slogan 'Don't Die of Ignorance', did little to alleviate it. Useful information about staying safe from infection was limited and confusion about HIV

transmission continued. A Gallup poll in March 1987 suggested that most people had found the Government's leaflet nowhere near explicit enough. Meanwhile AIDS helplines received calls from parents whose children had wanted to know what ignorance was and how you could avoid catching it.

If the advertisements were not illuminating, they were certainly frightening. Images such as the violent eruption of a phallic-looking volcano (presumably intended to signify how rapidly the virus might spread) and a gravestone with the word AIDS chiselled on it, made an obvious association between sex and death which had a powerful impact upon the imaginations of many.

Suddenly, doctors at sexually transmitted disease (STD) clinics were dealing with a massively increased demand for HIV antibody testing. The Public Health Laboratory Service reported a three-fold increase in tests carried out between November 1986 and March 1987, although the number of infected people recorded during that period increased at exactly the same rate as before. The vast majority of people that doctors were seeing for tests were HIV negative. Their tendency to interpret their anxiety about AIDS as the first symptoms of the condition itself led counsellors and medical practitioners to label them the 'worried well' of the HIV epidemic.

However, in one important respect the campaign had broken new ground. For the first time, the word 'condom' was mentioned in a television advertisement, though the authority of the special Cabinet AIDS Committee was required to approve this. It was not until 1 August 1987 that the ban on television publicity of condoms (which had been in existence for 27 years) was finally lifted, by which time the Independent Broadcasting Authority (IBA) had issued guidelines on the form such commercials should take. Condom ads had to be, for example, 'restrained and in good taste', show a sense of social responsibility, avoid promoting promiscuity, and, above all, not show the product 'unwrapped'.

IBA officials would certainly have baulked at the type of publicity condoms would receive elsewhere a year or two later. A 1989 television commercial by the French Health Ministry showed a naked couple reaching for a condom prior to having sex, and in Denmark government publicity in 1988 included television close-ups of a rubber being rolled down an erect penis. The first condom commercial in the UK – showing a young couple (fully clothed) meeting to embrace above the slogan 'together you're safer with Durex' – was tame viewing by comparison.

Despite the IBA restrictions, the condom industry flourished and continues to do so. Condoms in all colours, shapes, sizes, smells and tastes are now available; Japanese scientists have even produced a musical condom that plays the Beatles' hit *Love Me Do* when removed from its wrapper. In August 1991, *Condomania* - the first British shop to specialise in supplying condoms - opened its doors to the public. Its slogan? Whatever your condom needs, we've got you covered.

CARING IN A CRISIS

No apparent upsurge in the use of condoms, however, could prevent the immediate crisis health authorities were facing by early 1987, especially those in the London area where numbers of people with HIV were highest. Some health authorities were having to pay for AIDS care using money allocated for other purposes, and funds for *zidovudine*, the only drug licensed for treating people with AIDS in the UK (at a 1987 cost of £5,400 per patient per year), were running out.

At the same time, it was becoming apparent that effective care for people with HIV disease within the community would not be a cheap alternative to providing hospital beds. Following a six-day tour of HIV-related community care facilities in New York and San Francisco, Health Minister Norman Fowler announced a six-point programme for the UK, allowing nurses, family doctors and social workers to get experience of providing services that would allow people with HIV to be cared for in their own homes. It was only a starting point, but would cost around £250,000.

Meanwhile, the London Lighthouse, a centre for people with HIV and AIDS in west London which provides hospice, respite care and other facilities, was being financed almost entirely by the fundraising efforts of actors and celebrities like Elizabeth Taylor and Ian McKellen. The centre opened in 1988 and cost over £4 million to build; running costs in its first year were estimated at £1.5 million.

Services were urgently needed to slow the rapid increase of HIV infection among injecting drug users. In late 1986, the Scottish Committee on HIV had reported that as many as 50 per cent of injecting users in the east of Scotland were already infected. It was apparent that the risk of HIV infection to injecting drug users through shared equipment was becoming far more significant than any other risks posed by drug-taking. To make access to clean injecting equipment less problematic, the Government announced that 12 centres would be set up in hospitals and drug agencies where used needles and syringes could be exchanged for new ones.

Another outcome of the Minister's trip to the US was the decision to set up an umbrella organisation to coordinate the work of the voluntary sector in HIV, and to fund research. On 5 May 1987, the National AIDS Trust (NAT) was launched. It was to work closely with a body which, in the same year, had been given a new name and a new role in HIV education. The Health Education Council, an independent body which produced information and monitored health in the UK, was renamed the *Health Education Authority* (HEA) in March 1987 and took on the task of running HIV education campaigns for the Department of Health. In the process of so doing it lost its autonomy. This loss would, over the following years, increasingly hamper its ability to provide helpful and hard-hitting messages to the British public.

DECLARATION AGAINST DISCRIMINATION

1988 was declared by a world summit of Health Ministers to be a year of communication about AIDS. A meeting in London in early January resulted in an International Declaration on AIDS (known as *The London Declaration*), calling for the preservation of human rights and dignity for HIV-positive people, and avoidance of stigmatisation.

Although the declaration had no legally-binding status, as a statement of good intent it had significance. During discussion of discrimination, a number of delegates admitted that in their countries immigration laws and HIV antibody testing policy operated against HIV-positive foreigners requiring residence and nationals returning from work abroad.

In the UK, people with HIV were reported to have been sacked from their jobs because colleagues feared infection, and to have been refused accommodation or evicted from their homes if landlords heard (or made assumptions) about their HIV status. Life assurance companies were refusing to provide cover for people with the virus; some were even denying assurance to people who had taken the HIV antibody test, whatever the result might be. There was also worry about rejection and hostility from others. In London, there had been reports of people with AIDS having their homes burnt down by neighbours, or committing suicide because of the stigma attached to their condition.

The health ministers agreed that 'urgent action' was needed by governments to support the World Health Organization's newly established *Global Programme on AIDS*. A special day was set aside for remembering AIDS each year; December 1st, or World AIDS Day.

At the time of making this decision there were over 75,000 known cases of AIDS globally (the WHO considered the real figure to be nearer 150,000) and an estimated 5 to 10 million people with HIV. The epidemiologist Sir Richard Doll had expressed the view that the British HIV epidemic looked set to replace heart disease and lung cancer as the greatest threat to public health in the latter part of the twentieth century, a prediction which still looks likely today. He called for a new gauge for tracing the spread of the virus, in the form of 'routine screening' for HIV infection.

MEASURING THE EPIDEMIC

What he meant by routine screening (which later came to be known as anonymous screening) was that HIV antibody tests could be performed on patients' blood samples without their knowledge, and with all identifying information removed, so that those carrying out the tests would not know to whom the blood belonged. The theory was that the patient would thus avoid the trauma of a positive test result, while statisticians and health service planners would be provided with a clearer idea of the spread of HIV in the population.

In December of 1988, the Government was ready to carry this policy forward. It announced that a wide-scale anonymous screening programme would be set up, testing blood samples routinely collected from hundreds of thousands of people attending hospitals, sexually transmitted disease clinics and GPs' surgeries.

The decision followed several months of fiercely-argued debate about the practical value and ethical justification for such a programme. While organisations such as the HEA and the British Medical Association considered that a more wide-ranging approach than voluntary testing was necessary to produce accurate HIV prevalence data, others felt that mass surveillance of this sort would be ineffective, since a high proportion of the test results were likely to be HIV negative. Organisations such as the THT argued that a more urgent need might be to combat the risk of stigma and discrimination facing HIV-positive people. Until the Government recognised the need to legislate against such discrimination, a voluntary screening programme could never provide a complete picture of HIV prevalence in the UK.

A key aim of the anonymous screening programme was to find

out how fast HIV was spreading among heterosexuals. In 1988 a Government-appointed committee predicted between 10,000 and 30,000 new cases of AIDS would be diagnosed in the UK between 1987 and 1992, and between 7,500 and 17,000 deaths. The committee, which was chaired by Professor David Cox of Nuffield College, Oxford, thought that up to 50,000 people were already infected with HIV, and that the number of people with AIDS was being under-reported by as much as 20 per cent.

Although the Cox Committee's projections turned out to have erred on the side of pessimism – the rate of increase of new AIDS diagnoses actually slowed down between 1987 and the end of 1988 – this had little to do with the response of heterosexuals to the epidemic. Instead, it was widely considered to be due to sexual behaviour changes among gay men in the early to mid-1980s. The general view was that the epidemic among gay men was nearing its peak; among heterosexuals and injecting drug users, the opposite was true.

By the end of 1988, the percentage of women with HIV who had been infected through sex was shown to have increased from 11 per cent in 1985 to around 40 per cent. In that same year, a clinic in Edinburgh revealed that 49 per cent of its male and 55 per cent of its female drug-using clients were HIV positive. A report by the Advisory Committee on the Misuse of Drugs called for a change of policy among drug services so that HIV prevention, rather than abstinence from drugs, might be seen as a primary goal for users. It proposed that chemists should be encouraged to sell syringes, and that free condoms should be supplied to drug users and people in prison.

Of these proposals, the idea of supplying prisoners with condoms continues to be by far the most controversial. Under the law there are no private places in prisons, and 'homosexual acts' are only legal in private. So provision of condoms to inmates had always been refused by the Home Office on the grounds that it would encourage a criminal offence. While agencies working with prisoners were well aware that sex between men takes place 'inside' on a regular basis, they have no way of knowing the real extent of such activity. Without data to support the need for provision of condoms in prisons, the Home Office refuses to sanction the idea. A study published in July 1991 found 8 per cent of a sample of 370 male ex-prisoners had had sex with other men in prison. The Home Office still considers the study to have been too small, and says that further research is needed. Thus it has effectively blocked any movement for change. In the meantime, the number of prisoners with HIV infection - estimated at about 1 in 100 in 1988 - continues to increase.

BACKLASH OF COMPLACENCY

If 1988 had been viewed as the year of communication about AIDS, 1989 began with warnings from Dr Jonathan Mann, the Director of WHO's Global AIDS Programme, about a 'backlash of complacency' which he said was threatening the success of international campaigns for HIV prevention. At a London conference on Health, Law and Ethics, Mann stated that AIDS was no longer newsworthy for many journalists: coverage in the press had halved since 1987. Journalists were not the only people who had lost interest in AIDS. In January, there was a full-day parliamentary debate on the subject in the House of Commons, which only 12 MPs thought it worthwhile to attend.

Even more seriously, it was clear that important messages about the need for comprehensive information on sexual behaviour to back HIV education campaigns were being ignored at the highest level. The HEA proposed a national survey of sexual attitude and lifestyles which would investigate the behaviour of 20,000 people and cost around £750,000. Funding for it would come from the HEA itself, the Economic and Social Research Council and the DoH.

Although there had been no such study in the UK for some 20 years, there was nothing extraordinary about this proposal; other countries had given similar research high priority. What *was* extraordinary was the Government's delay in carrying forward the survey, and its eventual decision to abandon it. In October 1989 it was announced that then-Prime Minister Margaret Thatcher had vetoed the project because she saw it as intrusive and unnecessary. Researchers would need to look elsewhere for financial backing, or abandon the scheme altogether.

This decision was made in the face of strong evidence that the survey would have been well received. Pilot studies of 1,000 people showed that over 70 per cent of participants had responded positively to the idea. It is therefore hard to see the sense of such a move. Did the Prime Minister mean that she did not believe heterosexuals to be at risk from HIV? Or did she simply know that many heterosexuals ignored their own risks of infection, and therefore had no wish to cause offence (or lose potential votes) by disabusing them?

Even before the sex survey was scrapped, the HEA had shown itself to be increasingly hampered by its responsibility to Government officials. In June 1988, 10,000 copies of a teaching pack for schools had been shredded at the last minute (at a cost of £25,000) because the Department of Education and Science did not feel they had a strong enough moral message. In late 1989, a £2 million HEA television campaign for 16- to 30-year-olds, which would have carried the slogan 'condoms are hip', was postponed. Officials were unable to say when the advertisements might be shown.

By the end of 1989, it appeared that Dr Mann's warnings about the dangers of complacency towards the HIV epidemic were alarmingly accurate. The Special Cabinet AIDS Committee, in existence for barely three years, had been disbanded, and at the beginning of 1990 the AIDS Division at the HEA was to be closed down. Instead, HIV/AIDS would become part of the organisation's programme on sexual health. HEA Chief Executive Dr Spencer Hagard said that 'it was felt we were regarding AIDS as a special sort of area that was unique and had different problems to other health education topics, when that was not, in fact, the case.'

NO SEX PLEASE, WE'RE BRITISH

Pressure was being applied to minimise the risk of HIV infection to heterosexuals. The influence of right-wing groups, which linked a religious interpretation of sexual morality with a traditionalist stance on gender roles under the broad title of 'family' issues, were getting involved in HIV prevention work. A spokesperson and sponsor for one such group, Sir Reginald Murley of Family and Youth Concern, did little to further the cause of HIV prevention when in November 1989 he stated that 'in this country we are just not seeing this disease spreading heterosexually unless people get involved in rather odd practices or sleep around to an excessive degree, perhaps with the type of person from whom you might be likely to acquire a disease.'

The 'rather odd practices' obliquely referred to by Murley did not include vaginal penetration; Family and Youth Concern had made clear that it considered the vagina, unlike the anus, to provide 'an inefficient means of transmitting HIV'. These conclusions stand in bald contradiction to the carefully researched findings of doctors, statisticians and scientists. Director of the British Medical Association AIDS Foundation Dr John Dawson reported in early

1990 that cases of HIV infection among heterosexuals were rising more rapidly than those among gay men or injecting drug users. In the last six months of 1989, there had been a 20 per cent rise in infection among heterosexuals, compared with the 9.6 per cent rise among gay or bisexual men and 6.1 per cent among injecting drug users. It was becoming increasingly obvious that there is no particular 'type of person' from whom one can expect to become infected with HIV; or rather, any 'type' at all.

On December 1 (World AIDS Day) 1989 – the theme that year was youth – 60 students gathered at the Institute of Contemporary Arts in London to look at HIV education materials and discuss their views. The event, which was organised jointly by the THT and the NAT, included a chance to ask the Health Minister, Virginia Bottomley, questions about the Government's policy on AIDS. Members of the press were present, and the Minister was not let off lightly. One young man raised his hand to ask her a question.

'Am I right in thinking that the Government has been running public education campaigns on AIDS since 1986, Minister?' he asked.

'That is correct,' replied the Minister.

'Why then' said the young man, 'did none of them tell me that masturbation and oral sex could be fun and safe? Until I came here today, I thought safer sex was just screwing with a condom on.'

The Minister looked around the room for inspiration. Journalists scribbled frantically in their note pads. As one of them remarked in coverage of the event, Bottomley was certainly sitting in the hot seat.

ACTIONS, NOT WORDS

Abroad, as in the UK, HIV prevention initiatives had become heavily politicised. Dr Jonathan Mann, Director of the WHO's Global Programme on AIDS, resigned in March 1990 after disagreements with the WHO's Director General Dr Hiroshi Nakajima. The resignation was partly due to frustration over Nakajima's alleged delay in implementing key HIV projects. 'I couldn't be responsible for directing a programme of words rather than actions,' said Mann.

If Mann wanted action, 1990 was the right year for it. In June, the annual International AIDS Conference took place in San Francisco, and yet a large proportion of delegates with HIV were unable to attend it. Following the changes proposed to American immigration law by President Reagan in 1987, it had become illegal for a person with HIV to enter the US. HIV-positive people wishing to visit the States had to apply to the US embassy in their own country for a special waiver, which was generally granted for visitors on business only. However, even if a visa were obtained, it allowed its owner to be clearly identified as having HIV infection, eliminating any confidentiality regarding antibody status.

In protest, a boycott of the San Francisco conference was organised by voluntary bodies in the UK, including the Terrence Higgins Trust, Haemophilia Society and the Non-governmental Organisations' Consortium on AIDS.

The boycott was initially successful; by early 1990, it had international support at ministerial level and had received considerable publicity. Over 100 AIDS service organisations joined it, and their absence from the conference made its point. By January 1991 a proposal to remove the immigration restrictions was made to the US Government. Unfortunately, shortly before the proposal became law the US Government backed down due to pressure from right-wing groups. The restrictions remain. As a result, the seventh International AIDS Conference, which was scheduled to be held in Boston, will now take place in Amsterdam.

In the UK, the newly appointed Prime Minister John Major announced at the end of 1990 that a figure of £42 million would be made available as an out-of-court settlement for over 1,200 people with haemophilia who had been infected by HIV from contaminated American imports of Factor 8, a blood-clotting agent available on the National Health Service in the early 1980s. By October 1990, 210 of those people had developed AIDS, and 140 were already dead.

The announcement of this settlement followed the most widely-publicised and hard-fought campaign for compensation since the HIV epidemic had begun. It was about half of what could have been expected from a successful litigation, but was finally accepted by the majority of people with haemophilia, with what David Watters, General Secretary of the Haemophilia Society, described as 'a great deal of resignation'.

The high-profile campaign on the part of the Haemophilia Society had enjoyed the support of influential MPs, journalists and AIDS professionals. Press coverage was extremely high and generally sympathetic, possibly because a key issue of the campaign – that of state incompetence leading to individual suffering – could be seen to have a universal appeal.

Other campaigns cannot rely on such widespread support from the public and do not necessarily have the funds to put across their messages in sophisticated ways. Bodies such as ACT UP (the AIDS Coalition to Unleash Power) have regularly taken their anger onto the streets, organising marches, rallies and demonstrations on issues such as delays in trialling new drugs that might prolong the lives of people with HIV, or the under-representation of women and black people on drug trial volunteer groups. Since the late 1980s in the UK and the US, direct actions taken by HIV/AIDS activists have played an increasingly important role in campaigning for change.

A TIME OF TRIALS

In the US, a group of gay men, frustrated by the lengthiness of the testing and approval process of drugs going through federal trials, have set up a Community Research Initiative so that reliable information about useful drugs may be made available more rapidly. Volunteers with HIV are able to participate in experimental trials, which are ethically monitored so that no participant will receive a placebo (a harmless substance) instead of a potentially useful drug, unless this was what he or she wishes.

In the UK, an attempt to create a similar body has been unsuccessful. While a high proportion of Government research funds have been committed to developing a vaccine against HIV infection, organisations such as THT have argued that research into the development of drugs to prevent or delay illness in people who are already HIV positive has been relatively limited.

Zidovudine is still the only licensed treatment for people with HIV in the UK. However, in mid-1990 a new anti-viral treatment known as *dideoxyinosine*, or DDI, began trials in Britain. As with zidovudine, there is no assumption that DDI will be a 'cure' for HIV. However, for the one person in three with HIV for whom zidovudine has become dangerous or ineffective, it offers considerable hope of an improved quality of life.

The DDI trial, which runs parallel to one organised in France by INSERM, the French counterpart of the Medical Research Council (MRC), has broken important new ground in the way drug trials are organised within the UK. It allows participants to choose between getting a placebo or getting DDI at a high or low dose; previously volunteers had no choice in whether or not they were offered a placebo. It also allows participants to continue taking other drugs at the same time, and adopted a 'fast track' approach ~ which means that the required safety and effectiveness checks are implemented in half the time it normally takes for a new drug to reach trial stage.

FUN WITH FIGURES

Campaigners applying pressure for HIV treatments to be tested and made available more rapidly were becoming aware that they did not even have a clear idea of exactly how many people could benefit from such drugs. Anonymous screening to gain more accurate HIV prevalence data was taking time to produce results, and there were, in any case, a number of evident difficulties with the way in which HIV and AIDS statistics were being presented.

Since the late 1980s, AIDS workers had been complaining that the system used by the Communicable Diseases Surveillance Centre, which monitors and collates data on HIV and AIDS cases in England and Wales, was misleading and unhelpful. It made no consistent distinction between routes of infection and sexual identity, so that gay men with HIV were *always* assumed to have acquired the virus through sex with other men, while heterosexual men and women were subdivided into a range of categories depending on behaviour deemed to have caused infection. There were those who felt that such presentations obscured the extent of HIV infection among heterosexuals, particularly since there was an increasingly large number of 'undetermined' people who did not fit easily into any of the CDSC's categories and about whom no background information was available.

In early 1991, the CDSC's method of presenting HIV statistics finally changed, so that risky behaviour could be separated from social identity. For the first time also, the statistical presentations allowed a comparison of figures over a 12-month period, so that the rate of increase of infection through a specific route of transmission could be observed. This move aimed to make epidemiological analysis a little easier, and followed the launch on 22 October 1990 of a Public Health Laboratory Service AIDS Coordination Centre in North London, set up to improve surveillance and monitoring services in England and Wales.

AN EDUCATIONAL DILEMMA

Even if the presentation of HIV and AIDS figures had allowed some people to ignore the spread of HIV among heterosexuals, researchers had never ceased to be concerned. Heterosexual women in particular were at increasing risk. Studies suggested that the likelihood of a woman acquiring HIV through unprotected sex with a man in a regular sexual relationship was 1 in 4, compared with a 1 in 10 chance for a man becoming infected through an HIV-positive woman. The difference was attributed to trauma to the vagina during intercourse, cervical erosion and the absorbent properties of the vaginal walls, all of which might allow the virus to enter a woman's bloodstream.

In an interview for World AIDS Day 1990, the new Director of the WHO's Global AIDS Programme Dr Michael Merson said that an estimated 1 in 40 African women, 1 in 500 South American women and 1 in 700 North American women were infected with the virus. Globally, this amounted to some 3 million women with HIV infection.

By late January 1991 there was evidence that some young gay men were having unsafe sex with male partners their own age, the grounds that only gay men in their 30s and 40s were likely to be infected. Such findings may have prompted the Government's Chief Medical Officer Sir Donald Acheson to remark at an April conference on sexual health that efforts must be made in schools to 'introduce issues of heterosexuality and homosexuality at an even earlier age', to combat what he saw as an 'extraordinary ignorance about sexual behaviour and attitudes'.

These remarks were welcomed by those well-acquainted with the difficulties teachers face in tackling issues of sexuality and HIV with students. Section 28 of the Local Government Act 1987 makes it an offence for teachers to 'promote' homosexuality in the classroom (whatever that might mean), and although secondary schools are required by law to include AIDS education in their curriculum, under the Education Act 1986 school governors can decide to veto sex education if they so wish. A teacher might therefore be able to discuss sex, but not be able to give details about sexuality; or he or she may be allowed to teach about AIDS, but not necessarily about sex.

For gay men, it has become increasingly difficult to express sexuality at all without fear of recrimination. In the eyes of those who want homosexuality to be viewed as a criminal offence, Section 28 has not been enough. Under the Home Office's Criminal Justice Bill, soliciting by a man and what police judged to be 'indecency' between men can be turned into serious sex crimes (lesbians are not included; as far as some people are concerned, they do not exist).

From the late 1980s onwards, AIDS service organisations have worried that gay men would become more and more afraid to come forward for advice and help.

THE STRUGGLE FOR FUNDING

Nine years into the HIV epidemic, the most innovative and effective projects continue to be developed by charities and community groups. AIDS services run by the voluntary sector remain indispensable, and standards high, despite competition for grants, despite the stress, disillusionment and personality clashes engendered by a time of rapid expansion and change.

However, it is becoming more difficult to meet the demands of clients and retain funding for future initiatives. National Health Service changes have resulted in the emergence of a 'contract culture', where health authorities are expected to buy in services from other agencies. For organisations reliant on Department of Health funding, such as the London Lighthouse and Terrence Higgins Trust, this means that contracts need to be drawn up with dozens of different health authorities to secure the necessary funds in return for provision of services to a specified number of patients in each district. 'Accountability' is the buzzword used by ministers and MPs to justify the administrative overhaul; yet many already over-stretched AIDS service organisations have great difficulty finding the extra staff time and financial resources to make such accountability possible.

Voluntary bodies working in AIDS have always been under scrutiny, both because, as with other charities, a considerable proportion of their funding comes from public donations, and because there are still journalists who seek to prove that HIV is an issue for minority groups alone. Thus, the argument runs, such groups should cope on their own; money spent by those who do not belong in 'high-risk' categories on HIV prevention and care is effectively money down the drain.

A SILENT EPIDEMIC?

From the beginning, the struggle to limit the potentially devastating impact of HIV upon the health of the British public has been undercut by the terms in which success or failure have tended to be measured. If, in the early days of the epidemic, a growing level of infection among groups often seen as somehow outside the 'general population' could be ignored, who would decide what level of suffering would turn the HIV epidemic into an unacceptable problem that merited universal attention? While debate about HIV and AIDS in Parliament and the press focuses upon the notion of a 'heterosexual explosion', the relatively low (albeit increasing) rate of infection among heterosexuals in the UK is not considered dramatic enough by many to necessitate behaviour change.

Does an 'explosion' really have to take place before the message sinks in that *anyone* practising unsafe behaviour could be at risk? Even now, few people have any clear idea what such an 'explosion' might represent, but for AIDS educators it would mean that prevention messages were ineffective and had come far too late.

The HIV epidemic has been seen by many as a 'silent' one, largely unacknowledged in Britain (as in most countries) for years, until action to slow the spread of the virus and provide care for HIV-positive people became unavoidable. As Chapter 2 illustrates further, it is also regarded as a silent epidemic in the sense that people with the virus may be unaware that they are HIV positive and live without symptoms of infection. In some cases, they may never develop HIV-related illness, a prospect which looks increasingly likely as more effective preventive drug therapies become available.

Whether or not people are aware that they are HIV positive, they remain infectious to others. This might appear to make the prevention of HIV transmission impossible. However, preventing transmission depends on changing behaviour, not on knowing everyone's HIV status. There are considerable grounds for hope in such information, but the challenge presented is universal. If we confront it, the course of the 'silent' epidemic could radically change.

The chapters that follow explore HIV transmission in greater detail, and look at the possibilities of behaviour change for *everyone*, whether HIV negative or positive.

—— 2 ——

A Medical Condition

THE STRUCTURE OF HIV

HIV, or the *Human Immunodeficiency Virus* is, like all viruses, not a complete cell; it is made up of an inner core of genetic material enclosed in a protective envelope of protein.

Viruses cannot be said to be alive because they are unable to reproduce until they enter cells belonging to their host (in other words, the body they are occupying). This is part of the process of infection, and involves the virus injecting the 'host' cell with viral genetic material, so that the cell reproduces the virus.

Most organisms, including viruses, store a type of genetic 'blueprint' of themselves in the form of a chemical called Deoxyribonucleic acid (DNA), which contains the genetic code a virus needs to reproduce itself. This means that when a virus has attached itself to the host cell and inserted its own DNA into that cell, the cell is forced to reproduce new viral protein, which reassembles into viruses and bursts free from the host cell, often killing it in the process.

HIV is a *retrovirus*, the name given to a group of viruses which contain genetic material stored differently from other viruses. In retroviruses, the genetic material is stored in a chemical form called Ribonucleic acid (RNA). When a retrovirus enters a host cell, it forces the cell to make DNA from the viral RNA. This is contrary to what happens when a non-retrovirus infects a cell, because then the cell makes RNA from the viral DNA. This is why retroviruses are so named: 'retro' means backwards, and retroviruses operate in the opposite way to 'ordinary', non-retroviruses.

The types of retrovirus with which HIV is associated fall into two groups: *oncoviruses*, which are associated with cancers, and *lentiviruses*, so-called because they are slow (*lentus* in Latin) to act on the body. HIV is now considered to be a lentivirus, although

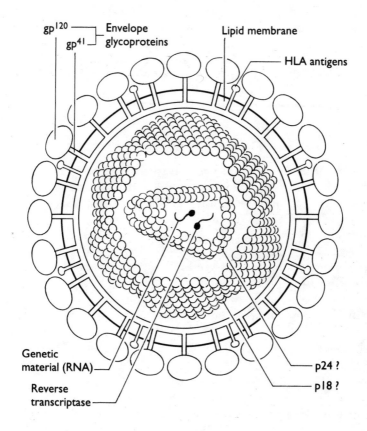

A model of the structure of HIV

early research linked it more closely with the oncovirus group, partly because cancer viruses frequently affect humans, whereas lentiviruses have hardly ever been shown to do so previously.

Drawings of HIV have represented the virus as a circle covered by an outer shell with little tentacles (representing molecules of protein on the coat of the virus) sticking out of it. Each virus is tiny – it has a diameter of only 0.1 micrometres, and a thousand million viruses stuck together would still be barely visible to the naked eye, measuring around one tenth of a millimetre across. On the outside of this viral envelope, the protein molecules (called *glycoproteins*) are spaced at regular intervals. HIV has two sorts of glycoprotein, called gp120 and gp41.

Inside this viral envelope there is a structure called the *core shell*, which is a layer probably made of a protein called p18. Inside the core shell is the core of the virus, in which the genetic material of HIV, the RNA, is contained. The core also holds an enzyme called *reverse transcriptase*, which scientists believe helps HIV to turn its RNA into DNA and then insert its DNA into that of the host cell. *How HIV Infects the Cells of the Immune System*, below, explains this in more detail.

Different Strains of HIV

HIV, like other viruses, changes its structure slightly each time it reproduces (a process called *mutation*), so that the body's immune system has difficulties recognising it. Sometimes this results in very distinct strains of the virus emerging, which may help to explain the variations in the way HIV-related illness develops in people in different geographical areas.

This variation in experience of HIV illness can make it difficult to distinguish between strains of the same virus and a different type of virus altogether. To date, numerous strains of HIV have been identified, but only two different basic virus types: HIV1 (often called just HIV) and HIV2. HIV2 was first discovered in two people with AIDS from West Africa in 1986, and it has spread rapidly there since. It has also now been reported in the United States and Europe; it was first reported in Britain in 1988.

Globally, HIV2 is considered to be far less common than HIV1, and is thought to be much more closely linked with a monkey virus – *Simian Immunodeficiency Virus* (SIV) – than with HIV1. Its genetic material and structure is different from that of HIV1, and researchers consider that it may remain dormant in the body much longer than HIV1 does. It is also possible that people with AIDS caused by the virus HIV2 may survive longer with the condition, but little is known about this, or about the number of people who may be infected with both HIV1 and HIV2.

In early 1988, researchers claimed to have identified a third member of the HIV family, HIV3, but as no further developments have been reported since then, it appears likely that what was identified as HIV3 was simply another strain of HIV1 or HIV2. Scientists have also claimed to have isolated a third form of HIV in fluids drawn from the brain, but as yet there is no strong evidence to support their view.

HIV1 and HIV2 may differ in their biological properties, but, like all forms of HIV, they do not differ in the ways in which they are transmitted. Both can also be destroyed easily when outside the body through infection control measures such as the use of heat and disinfectants. This is important, because although viral variation makes it more difficult to develop a vaccine that will recognise all the different types of HIV, we can at least be sure that once we know how to stay safe (or, if HIV positive, how to protect others from the virus), that information will continue to serve us well.

THE HUMAN IMMUNE SYSTEM

Our body's defence against infections has two key components: our skin, which forms a protective barrier against harmful elements outside that could damage us, and our immune system, which is based on the complex processes of a range of cells and molecules in our blood. (Scientists sometimes refer to this as *cell-mediated immunity*.)

The immune system has the job of recognising and getting rid of foreign substances (or *antigens*) that have already entered the body. Antigens can be any type of foreign material: a cancer cell, a transplanted organ, or the protein coat of a virus or bacterium. The body encounters numerous antigens daily, and disposes of most of them quickly, although sometimes (possibly because it has not come across a particular antigen before) the immune system does not operate quickly enough, and the infection takes over. Gradually however, the body mounts a response to the infection by producing *antibodies*, or protein molecules that seek out and stick to particular antigens in an attempt to eliminate them.

The workings of the immune system are complex and incompletely understood, but there are two key groups of blood cells in operation: *phagocytes* and *lymphocytes*. Phagocytes swallow up and destroy antigens. They consist of large cells called *macrophages*, which engulf and destroy bacteria and some viruses, and *monocytes*, smaller, immature forms of cell that can turn into macrophages if necessary. Macrophages and monocytes are initially produced in the bone marrow, but are later located throughout a person's body.

Lymphocytes are considered to be crucial in controlling the way the body deals with infections. Cells called *B lymphocytes*, or *B-cells* are responsible for producing antibodies which stick to invading micro-organisms and either inactivate them at once, or make it easier for other cells to do this.

T lymphocytes, or *T-cells* play a number of different roles. *T-suppressor cells* work by suppressing the immune system's response to infection, when appropriate. They are able to prevent B-cells from producing antibodies indefinitely once the infection is under control. *T-cytotoxic cells* (sometimes called T 'killer' cells) attack infected cells to stop the organisms inside them from reproducing and spreading the infection further. *T-helper cells* supervise the operation, regulating the activity of B-cells, suppressor and cytotoxic T-cells, and macrophages, alerting them to the presence of an intruder. They are also able to send the immature cells, or monocytes, to places of infection, where these can develop into macrophages and engulf invading antigens.

It is these T-helper cells that seem to be most severely affected by HIV infection; in a person with AIDS, there is an acute shortage of these cells, while in a healthy person there are more T-helper cells than either cytotoxic or suppressor T-cells.

How HIV Infects the Cells of the Immune System

The process by which HIV infects a cell can perhaps be most clearly understood as a series of steps, as outlined below.

1. 'Locking on' to the Cell

Once HIV is inside the bloodstream, it has to stick to the surface of cells in order to enter them. It is thought that the virus does this by 'locking on' to the outside membrane of a cell. This is thought to occur when the glycoprotein gp120, located on the envelope of the virus, sticks to a molecule on the outside of some cells, called CD4. It is still not clear what triggers the initial binding process, nor what exactly occurs at the junction of cell and virus. Sometimes it appears that HIV can 'lock on' to a cell without invading it afterwards.

There are three types of cell in the immune system which carry the CD4 molecule: T-helper cells, B-cells, and macrophages. While T-helper cells and B-cells may be invaded, and later destroyed by infection with HIV, it appears that this does not occur with macrophages. Instead, macrophages are thought to carry HIV with them as they circulate through the body, releasing and therefore spreading the virus as they go. In other words, they may act as a type of 'mobile container' for the virus.

2. Inserting Viral Genetic Material into that of the Cell

Once it is attached to the cell, the virus inserts its genetic material (RNA) into that cell, with the viral enzyme *reverse transcriptase*. Inside the cell, the reverse transcriptase enzyme turns the RNA of HIV into DNA. This newly-produced viral DNA is now a complete genetic code for HIV. In order to make the cell it has invaded reproduce more HIV, the DNA of the virus has next to be integrated into the DNA of the cell.

It may be helpful to imagine this as a string of beads which fit into each other (the DNA of the cell) being forced apart and new beads (the viral DNA) inserted to make another string. The cell will now contain the genetic material of HIV throughout its lifetime.

3. Lying Low

The viral DNA may stay in the cell for a long time without reproducing. This is sometimes called a *dormant* or *latent* period, and means that a person with HIV may live for years without developing symptoms of illness. It is still uncertain whether the majority of people with HIV infection will become ill at all, although current research suggests that about 50 per cent of people with HIV develop related illness within 10 years of the date of infection.

During the latent period, the body is likely to respond to infection by producing antibodies, as it does with any infection from an invading organism. It may take the cells of the immune system as little as three weeks after infection to produce antibodies to HIV, or it may take several months (in very rare cases it may take a year or more). Most people develop antibodies to HIV in three to six months' time, and the process is called *seroconversion*, because the blood has changed from having no antibodies to HIV infection to having them.

What is important is that the antibodies produced to get rid of HIV *do not seem to work*. They do not prevent the virus from hiding in the cells of the body's immune system and causing damage to it later on. It is not clear why this is so. Some researchers suggest that the body does not produce enough antibodies to deal with the infection, or that the antibodies are not up to the job. Other theories include the idea that not everybody produces antibodies, and that the people who don't therefore become ill eventually. It is also possible that the antibodies are effective for a long time (while the virus is inactive in the body) but later on production of antibodies stops, so the immune system is overcome by the virus.

Antibodies are not the only response of the body to invasion by HIV. It seems likely that the T-cytotoxic or 'killer' cells also attack the virus, and some scientists see this as a more effective

41

response to HIV infection than the production of antibodies. Research has shown that people with HIV with symptoms of related illness have low levels of these T-cytotoxic cells, which may mean that many of the cells have tried to 'mop up' HIV, have become infected with the virus, and have died.

4. Activation of HIV

HIV may be dormant in cells for a long period of time, then begin to reproduce itself. Even during the dormant phase of infection, the virus may be actively reproducing in some cells, but at such low levels that no changes are caused in the health of the infected person.

One possible reason for HIV being activated in the invaded cells is that those cells are being stimulated by the presence of another foreign antigen. Another theory is that HIV is triggered into action when the DNA of the invaded cell interacts with the genetic material of another virus also invading that cell.

Once the DNA of a cell is activated, it turns into a sort of 'factory' for the production of new particles of HIV. The HIV particles travel to the surface of the cell and burst out of it, taking parts of the cell's membrane with them and using this to form the envelope for new viruses. The cell is likely to explode and die in the process of producing new viruses. Meanwhile, the new viruses are released into the blood and can join up with more blood cells, starting the process of infection all over again.

THE HIV ANTIBODY TEST

Although often referred to mistakenly as the 'AIDS test', the HIV antibody test cannot tell you whether or not you have any sort of HIV illness, or whether you are likely to become ill in the future.

The test works by detecting antibodies to HIV infection in the bloodstream. If antibodies are found to be present, the test result is said to be 'positive', and the person whose blood is being tested is considered to have been exposed to HIV infection (to be 'HIV positive' or 'seropositive'). If antibodies are not found to be present, the test result is said to be 'negative', and the person concerned is considered not to have HIV infection (to be 'HIV negative' or 'seronegative').

Deciding whether or not to take the HIV antibody test is not necessarily an easy matter. Much more detailed information is given in Chapter 6 about how the test works, how it is used, and what the advantages and disadvantages of taking the test may be for any individual.

HIV ILLNESS

The information below focuses on the symptoms and diseases that may occur during the course of HIV infection. It may well be of use for people with HIV who want further information about the specific illnesses they have and the treatments they may be receiving. Chapter 7 gives more detailed information about other aspects of living with HIV.

It is always worth getting further information from other sources (see the Directory at the back of this book for relevant publications and organisations), as news about drug therapies is constantly in need of updating. The information given here is accurate at the time of writing.

If you think that what follows may lead you to diagnose yourself as having a disease of any sort, you might want to think twice about reading it. You cannot make decisions about your health on the basis of what is said here. If you have any worries about illness, you need to seek help and advice from trained professionals.

Mistaken Labels?

Early on in the HIV epidemic, doctors and scientists decided to regard infection with the virus as a series of stages of illness. These are defined by the state of a person's immune system and symptoms of disease: they range from the short-term illness which sometimes follows infection to the final development of what was called AIDS.

However, it is unlikely that an idea of carefully labelled stages of infection is helpful in the long term, either to doctors or people living with HIV. As stated in Chapter 1, it is quite possible to die from HIV-related illness without having an AIDS diagnosis. Similarly, even though it has a precise medical definition, AIDS is diagnosed and experienced in very different ways globally, depending on geographical location, prevalent infections in the region of diagnosis, and resources available for treatment and care.

What is now also evident is that there is no clear-cut chronological progression between the neatly-labelled stages of infection. It is possible to go from being healthy with HIV to a diagnosis of AIDS, by-passing the stages in between. Similarly, it seems to be possible to have HIV infection without becoming ill at all, or to reach different stages of infection without developing AIDS, or to move backwards and forwards between phases, so that a person may have symptoms of illness at one point and then feel healthy again. For these reasons, the phrase 'HIV illness' is now increasingly used as an umbrella term to describe any degree of HIV-related illness.

Despite the fact that these rather artificially defined stages of infection are increasingly redundant, they are still regularly used by doctors, statisticians, researchers and journalists. Elsewhere in this book I have used the term 'AIDS' because it is still seen as a relevant indicator of advanced HIV illness. Where it is used it is meant generally in the sense of a statistical marker: for some years now, epidemiologists have used AIDS cases as a yardstick for the development of the HIV epidemic. Where information given applies generally to people with *any* degree of HIV-related disease (including what is clinically defined as AIDS), I have preferred to use the term 'HIV illness'.

In fact, we are probably stuck with the AIDS label until doctors and scientists agree that HIV infection should be seen in a more flexible way, allowing not just for the possibility of continuous progression between stages of increasing illness, but also for the idea of recovery and restoration of the immune system. Until this happens, it may be wise to be informed about the idea of clearly defined stages of infection, since HIV is still measured by some people in that way.

At the same time, HIV-positive people may need to be familiar with the notion that living with HIV means coping with what may seem to be a massive contradiction. This is the result of the combination of extreme uncertainty about the course of infection and the extraordinary degree to which individuals can control their health and recover quickly from disease when it occurs.

In the following section a dual approach has been taken. There is a brief discussion about 'stages' of HIV infection, but also information about different symptoms and illnesses, in no particular chronological order. Instead, they are arranged in order of the part of the body they affect: where an antigen may affect different areas of the body they are cross-referenced.

Illnesses occurring as a result of the body's damaged immune system through HIV infection are often called 'opportunistic' infections. Where there are drugs to treat or prevent these, brief details of some of the key treatments are given under the relevant infection.

The Theoretical Phases of HIV Infection

Acute Infection with HIV

Many people who have just become infected with HIV will have no physical symptoms of ill health. On the other hand, others may experience a brief period of illness. Symptoms tend to be varied but might include feeling 'fluey', running a temperature, tiredness, aches and pains, and possibly a skin rash. This brief period around the date of infection is called the *acute* period of infection; none of the symptoms of illness at this early stage are long-lasting or serious, except in very rare cases. It is also important to remember that these symptoms *on their own* do not constitute a diagnosis of HIV infection. Unless you have received a positive HIV antibody test result (see above), you cannot make assumptions on the basis of such symptoms. Ordinary stress and fatigue, glandular fever or flu, for example, often have the same kind of effect upon your health as does the acute phase of HIV infection.

Chronic Asymptomatic Infection

In many people with HIV, the acute infection stage is followed by a long period of good health. This is called the period of *chronic* (or lasting) infection, and varies in length between each individual. It is an *asymptomatic* phase, because people at this stage do not show symptoms of HIV illness. This is another area where there are still large uncertainties: it is generally difficult, if not impossible, to know whether an asymptomatic person with HIV will stay healthy or not. Some adults may receive an AIDS diagnosis just a few months after the date of exposure to the virus, while others may not become ill for ten years or more, if at all.

While scientists estimate that an adult with HIV aged less than 60 years has a 50 per cent chance of developing AIDS within 7 to 10 years from the date of infection, such statistics are nothing more than informed guesses. It is very important to stress that HIV infection may not necessarily lead eventually to illness and death.

The factors that may contribute to triggering illness in a person with HIV are also incompletely understood. However, the age of the person concerned is relevant. Babies born with HIV infection may be diagnosed as having AIDS when they are only six months old, because the immune system of a very young child tends to be weaker than that of an adult, and therefore less able to deal with infection (see *Children and HIV Illness*, below). Similarly, old age may make the period of chronic infection shorter.

The general level of fitness of a person with HIV is also important. A person in good health is likely to stay well for longer with HIV infection than someone who is in poor health prior to infection. Poor diet, lack of sleep, severe stress and the presence of other infections in the body are also considered significant factors in the development of HIV disease. In general, it is thought that there is a great deal a person with HIV can do to protect his or her health and live as well as possible with the virus; Chapter 7 gives more information about this.

Persistent Generalised Lymphadenopathy (PGL)

As people with HIV infection may develop swollen lymph glands for prolonged periods, this condition has been described as *persistent generalised lymphadenopathy*, or PGL. PGL usually involves swellings of lymph glands in the neck to a diameter of 1 cm or more. Swollen lymph glands may also occur in the groin, but are not considered a symptom of PGL because they may be related to infections other than HIV. PGL is diagnosed when the swollen glands in the neck last for three months or more and cannot be related to any infection other than HIV. They are quite likely to be painless and invisible, although it is possible to feel them. They may also fluctuate in size.

AIDS-related Complex (ARC)

This is possibly the most nebulous and unhelpful of all categories of HIV infection, and the term is now in decreasing use. The ARC label has tended to apply to any type of HIV-associated illness that is not recognised as PGL or AIDS. It is therefore hopelessly broad and, in medical terms, largely meaningless.

The other problem with the use of this term is that people diagnosed with ARC may assume that they have 'reached the end of the road' – next there is AIDS, then death. This sense of an inevitable progression through increasingly severe illness presents a limited and undermining picture.

An AIDS Diagnosis

This is generally given to people with HIV infection, whose immune system is shown to be severely weakened, and who have one or more of a range of recognised diseases. As stated above, the illnesses that are taken as common indicators of AIDS across the world vary from one region to another, and among different social groups. AIDS diagnoses are, nevertheless, dependent on standards set by the American Centers for Disease Control (CDC).

Some medical conditions in people with HIV that would link with a diagnosis of AIDS are set out below.

- Protozoal infections, such as *cryptosporidiosis* (with diarrhoea for over a month), *pneumocystis carinii pneumonia*, and *toxoplasmosis*, which affects the brain.
- Fungal infections, such as *candidiasis* (thrush) and *cryptococossis*.
- Bacterial infections, such as *mycobacterium tuberculosis* (TB or related infections).
- Viruses, such as *herpes simplex* and *cytomegalovirus* disease.
- Cancers or malignancies, such as *Kaposi's sarcoma* and *lymphoma*.
- Other diseases include HIV *encephalopathy* (or dementia) and HIV *wasting disease* – unintentional excessive weight loss.

(The information above is borrowed with kind permission from the National HIV Prevention Information Service; Information File, July 1990.)

BEING HIV SYMPTOMATIC

The symptoms, infections and drug treatments described in the rest of this chapter do not make up a comprehensive list, but they do present a picture of some of the illnesses a person who is HIV symptomatic might experience in Britain. It should be stressed that where drug treatments are mentioned, this does not necessarily imply a recommendation.

For space reasons, the list is selective, but the most appropriate treatment for a person with HIV illness is a highly individual matter, and is best discussed with an experienced medical practitioner. In any case, information about HIV drugs under research and new treatments is constantly changing. The best way to stay really up to date is by reading some of the excellent newsletters on drug treatments available from the US and elsewhere, and by contacting relevant HIV organisations (see the Directory at the back of this book for details). Information on alternative medicine is given in Chapter 7.

The infections listed below apply in many cases to both women and men. However, it has been necessary to include separate sections on illnesses specific to women and children with HIV, in which areas information is still limited.

Severe Weight Loss

Excessive, unintentional weight loss in a person with HIV infection is sometimes called 'HIV wasting disease'. It can be caused by a range of factors, such as loss of appetite through drug treatments, anxiety or depression, stomach or mouth problems, inadequate ability to absorb food through bowel infections, or even a speeding up of the body's metabolism as it tries to deal with HIV-related infections.

In countries where diagnostic and treatment resources are scarce, severe and inexplicable weight loss may be the first signal of HIV infection. For this reason, in Africa AIDS is often referred to as 'Slim'.

Treatment
There is no obvious treatment for severe weight loss. While a doctor can help treat oral infections or diarrhoea, it may also help to get advice from a dietitian about vitamin supplements and nutritious high-calorie foods that are easy to digest.

Sweats and Fevers

Heavy sweating (particularly at night) and high temperatures are the usual response a body makes to viral infection. However, in the case of a person with HIV, they may also be an indicator of an opportunistic infection. A painkiller such as aspirin may help (but note that paracetamol is not appropriate for someone taking *zidovudine* – see below). It is also important to drink lots of fluids to replace the water lost through severe sweating.

Premature Ageing

People with HIV-related immune deficiency may experience symptoms of premature ageing, such as thinning skin and hair, 'going grey', and weight loss. Unfortunately, there are no cures for these symptoms, but the kind of basic guidelines for self-help given in Chapter 7 may be helpful in minimising the effects of ageing caused by recurrent infections and immune deficiency.

Chest Infections

Pneumocystis carinii pneumonia (PCP)
This is caused by a tiny organism that affects the lungs and hampers

the transfer of oxygen and carbon dioxide to and from the bloodstream. Most people are thought to be infected with *pneumocystis carinii* at some stage during childhood, but the infection very rarely appears to cause disease in people with healthy immune systems. It was first identified in patients with cancer undergoing deliberate immunosuppression in order to have organ transplants.

PCP is generally associated with quite severe immune deficiency, and was the first infection to draw HIV illness to doctors' attention in the United States in 1981. How the micro-organism is transmitted is uncertain, but in people with a weakened immune system it can be very serious, although the likelihood of mortality during a bout of PCP has fallen from around 30 per cent to about 12 per cent with improved medical knowledge and care. Unfortunately, co-factors such as having another lung infection at the same time, or it being a second attack of PCP may reduce the chance of recovery in a person with HIV.

Symptoms of PCP include a dry persistent cough, shortness of breath, fevers, sweats and weight loss. PCP can be fatal if untreated, and is an extremely common disease in people with AIDS; around 75 per cent are estimated to develop PCP at some point.

Treatment

Drugs to prevent and treat PCP are increasingly available. These include *septrin*, which tends to be given intravenously at first, then by mouth for three weeks. Septrin has been in use for PCP for some time, and can be effective against other bacteria present. However, it can have side-effects such as nausea or rashes in around 50 per cent of people with PCP.

Pentamidine is often given as a daily drip to people who experience side-effects with septrin. However, it has recently become possible to dispense pentamidine through a nebuliser or aerosol. This means that the drug is inhaled as a fine mist, and affects the lungs only. Early research indicates a significant degree of success with this method of taking pentamidine for people with mild PCP.

Prevention

Prevention of PCP (or *prophylaxis*) has become a significant issue for symptomatic people with HIV. There is still much research to be done in this area, but septrin used at lower doses than for treatment can be helpful in preventing PCP, as can nebulised pentamidine on the basis of an inhalation about once every two weeks. Nebulisers cost about £120, but the inhalation can be given free in hospital.

Pulmonary tuberculosis, or TB in the Lungs

This is caused by the mycobacterium of that name and is becoming increasingly prevalent in people with HIV. Symptoms of tuberculosis are coughs, fevers, shortness of breath and night sweats. It may also cause severe fatigue. In developing countries, where TB may be already latent in the population, it has become one of the most common HIV-related infections; it is also becoming more noticeable among injecting drug users in the United States. In Britain, there was an increase of TB in 1988, although it is not certain that this was due to HIV infection. People who have HIV and have previously been infected with TB may experience a reactivation of the condition, often with more severe illness and a higher mortality rate than those with TB who do not have immune deficiency.

Infection with mycobacterium tuberculosis can also cause illness outside the lungs, and this is so rarely seen in people who do not have HIV infection that the American Centers for Disease Control revised the 1985 standard definition of AIDS to include it in 1987. TB infection outside the lungs may lead to diarrhoea, weight loss and malnutrition.

Treatment

A range of drugs are used to treat pulmonary TB, often because mycobacterium tuberculosis may become resistant to one drug very easily. They include *rifampicin, isoniazid* and *streptomycin/amikacin*. These drugs are not without side-effects, however: rifampicin and isoniazid can both cause nausea and sometimes liver reactions. Generally drugs for TB have to be taken for a long time, because the bacterium can lie dormant in the lungs.

MAI

MAI, or *mycobacterium avium intracellulare*, is like TB, but requires a much greater degree of immune suppression (other mycobacteria of a similar sort are *mycobacterium kansasii* and *mycobacterium xenopii*, which are widespread but only appear to cause illness in people with severe immunosuppression). MAI is found in soil and tapwater, and can probably not be passed from one person to another. It causes lung problems but can also lead to diarrhoea, liver reactions, fever and weight loss.

Treatment
MAI is resistant to antibiotics, and drug treatments for it are limited.

- Pneumonias related to bacterial infection commonly lead to chest complaints in people who do not have immune deficiency, but in people with HIV these tend to be more prevalent. They may be caused by bacteria such as *haemophilus influenzae*, and symptoms include difficulties with breathing, coughs and pain in the lungs. As with mycobacterium tuberculosis, they can also lead to gastro-intestinal infections, causing weight loss and diarrhoea.
- Infections that occur fairly commonly in other parts of the body are also known to have an effect on the lungs from time to time. *Cytomegalovirus*, or CMV (see below), can cause inflammation in conjunction with PCP, and the fungus *Candida Albicans* also affects the lungs in rare cases. *Toxoplasma gondii* and Kaposi's sarcoma have also caused chest infections, although this is not their usual site of infection (see below).

Skin Conditions

The skin is a very common site for HIV-related infections. However, skin complaints are also common in HIV-negative people. Finding that you have developed dry skin, a fungal infection under a toe or fingernail or a series of warts are *not* adequate grounds to diagnose yourself with symptomatic HIV infection.

Kaposi's Sarcoma, or KS
This is a cancer that most commonly affects cells of the skin, but also the lungs, intestines and lymph nodes. On the skin it appears as purple patches which are sometimes slightly raised and generally painless, if disfiguring. KS in the lungs leads to chest infections and causes swelling in the lymph nodes due to the collection of fluid there. In the intestines it may lead to inability to absorb nutrients properly, causing bleeding and diarrhoea.

KS was first noticed in elderly Jewish men from Eastern European or Italian backgrounds with healthy immune systems, long before HIV was discovered. It is becoming less common in people with HIV generally, but has in any case been almost entirely confined to gay and bisexual men; HIV-positive women, children, people with haemophilia, injecting drug users and others rarely experience KS. The reasons for this are still unclear.

Treatment

Although KS is used as a diagnostic marker for AIDS, people with KS do not necessarily have severely depleted immune systems. Some people with KS stay healthy for a period of months or years, and KS can also disappear if the immune system recovers, following a kidney transplant, for example. However, some people with KS find the skin lesions disfiguring, particularly if they appear on the face, and so treatment options include cosmetic camouflage techniques and radiotherapy.

Drugs like *vincristine*, *vinblastine* and *bleomycin* can be injected into the lesion, or directly into the vein. As this has an effect upon the entire body and the drugs involved may have strong side-effects, it is only suitable for people with severe KS. It is generally only used in people with KS in internal organs, such as the lungs. *Alpha interferon* may restore some people's immune function to the point of clearing up KS, although this can be unpleasant to take and is by no means 100 per cent safe; by stimulating the immune system it may also stimulate the action of HIV on the body.

Shingles

This is a common infection among adults generally, but far more so among people with HIV-related illness. It results from infection with the *herpes zoster virus*, also called the *herpes varicella-zoster virus*. This is the virus that can cause chickenpox in children, after which it lies dormant in the body and may recur in adults (whether or not they have HIV infection) who are under severe stress. Herpes zoster virus causes a painful, itchy rash which can affect only one side of the body. If the rash involves the surface of the eye it can be serious, causing blindness. An adult with HIV-related immune deficiency who has never had chickenpox (and therefore has no natural immunity to herpes zoster) should probably avoid contact with a child with chickenpox, as this could lead to shingles.

The Herpes Simplex virus

Like herpes zoster, this can lie dormant in the body and be reactivated in people with weakened immune systems through HIV infection or other causes. Herpes simplex is often reactivated as cold sores, mouth or nostril spots, or, if acquired through sex, painful ulcers on the genitals and anus. Infection with herpes viruses can cause increased weakening of the immune system. The presence of genital ulcers caused by herpes simplex can make it easier to get HIV infection through unsafe sex. HIV-related herpes generally causes larger ulcers and lasts longer than in people who do not have HIV infection.

Treatment
Acyclovir is used both to treat herpes infections as a cream, pills or drip, and as a prophylactic measure for HIV symptomatic people, using a very low dosage.

Warts
These are relatively common conditions that tend to be seen more frequently in people with HIV. The wart virus, or *human papillomavirus*, causes warts which, in people with a damaged immune system, can become large and discoloured. In women, the wart virus has been linked with cervical cancer (see *Women and HIV Illness*, below). Warts around the anus in women and gay men with HIV can be acquired through anal sex, and may lead to a greater risk of anal cancer.

Treatment
Warts should be treated promptly by a medical practitioner using liquid nitrogen, podophyllin or heat treatment. Anti-wart medications from the chemist should be avoided, as they may irritate.

Skin funguses
Other skin infections such as athlete's foot or crotch, ringworm and seborrhoeic dermatitis, are all caused by funguses. They are present on everyone's skin, but only flare up in people with damaged immune systems or if the skin is moist and warm.

Treatment
Fungal infections can lead to flaky red skin, spots or dandruff, but can be treated by antifungal cream or pills. Keeping the skin dry and avoiding stress may also help.

Diseases of the Nervous System

Illness caused by the direct action of HIV or related infections upon the human nervous system is an emotive and difficult area. In the early stages of the HIV epidemic, people whose nervous system was damaged as a result of HIV infection tended to be diagnosed with 'AIDS dementia'. However, this term is probably unhelpful both because of the negative associations it has and because one general label blurs important distinctions between the complex range of infections that may cause neurological symptoms in people with HIV.

There is now reasonable evidence that most people with severe immune deficiency will develop some sort of disease of the nervous system, to a greater or lesser degree. However, it is very important to remember that psychological reactions to powerful events – such as a diagnosis of HIV infection or AIDS – can have short-term effects very similar to those seen in some people with neurological disease. For example, the initial symptoms of HIV encephalopathy, such as forgetfulness and an inability to concentrate, are a feature in the lives of many people who are fatigued or under pressure. Chapter 7 gives more information about dealing with stress relating to HIV infection.

HIV encephalopathy, or brain disease

This is caused by inflammation of the brain leading to impaired mental functions. It results from the direct action of HIV upon the brain cells, which, like T4 cells in the blood stream, have the CD4 receptor molecule onto which HIV locks itself. Nerve cells throughout the body also have the CD4 molecule, so HIV can lead to other conditions of the nervous system (see below).

Brain disease can occur in people with HIV shortly after they have become infected. This may last about a week and can cause fever, confusion, mood changes and fits. Symptoms are, however, generally thought to be temporary at this stage, and the anti-viral drug *zidovudine* (see below) is considered to be helpful in reversing such disease.

HIV encephalopathy, like KS, may occur at any stage of HIV infection. Unfortunately, when it does occur, the damage to the brain is usually permanent. Symptoms of HIV encephalopathy are likely to be fairly subtle initially, becoming more severe if the disease progresses. They might range from mild but repeated forgetfulness to difficulty walking and talking, failure to recognise people, and incontinence.

Treatment

At present, treatment for HIV encephalopathy is mainly through zidovudine, but it is hoped that other anti-viral drugs being trialled at present may be helpful. People with this disease can also make life easier for themselves by writing important things down whenever possible so that they don't have to carry details of appointments and so on in their heads. Keeping a diary may help, as may getting adequate rest and easing up on work in whichever ways are possible.

HIV peripheral neuropathy and autonomic neuropathy

These are diseases resulting from infection of nerve cells by HIV.

HIV peripheral neuropathy can occur when nerves throughout the body are affected; symptoms include numbness or weakness of limbs, difficulty in urination or incontinence, and sharp pain in the feet and hands.

Autonomic neuropathy is caused when the nerves controlling blood flow to internal organs are damaged by HIV. Symptoms include diarrhoea, dizziness and sexual impotence (although of course these can also be caused by other infections, or psychological factors such as stress).

Treatment

As yet there is no specific treatment for the neuropathy, but painkillers (see below), foot massage and the advice of a chiropodist can help.

There is no treatment specifically for autonomic neuropathy, but diarrhoea can be helped by drugs such as *imodium* and *codeine* and resultant dehydration through *rehydration therapy*. Dizziness may be alleviated by drugs like *fludrocortisone* or *hydrocortisone*.

Toxoplasma gondii

This micro-organism commonly affects adults when they eat infected, under-cooked meat. It is a widespread organism to which many people have been exposed; it multiplies in the intestines of cats and is found in cat-litter trays. Women who develop symptoms of toxoplasmosis for the first time during pregnancy are thought to have a 40 per cent chance of passing the infection to their babies in the uterus, and in around 10 per cent of the babies infected this way (called *congenital toxoplasmosis*) there may be severe brain damage. This has important implications for pregnant women with HIV, who may be more prone to toxoplasmosis as a result of immune deficiency.

For most adults with a healthy immune system, toxoplasma gondii does not produce symptoms of disease. However, in people with HIV, toxoplasmosis can cause abscesses in the brain which squash other brain tissues and result in severe headaches, confusion, fever and occasionally fits. Other effects may be loss of co-ordination, difficulty speaking and thinking, and numbness in one side of the body as a result of nerve destruction. Left untreated, the abscess may grow, possibly resulting in coma and finally death.

Treatment
Toxoplasmosis is, however, relatively easy to treat. Drugs such as *clindamycin* (in tablets or given intravenously), *maloprim* in tablet form, and *fansidar*, which can be administered as a drip or as tablets, are generally effective therapies, although not without side-effects.

Cryptococcus neoformans
This is a fungus that can cause *meningitis*, or infection around the brain, which can spread to other parts of the body. Symptoms of meningitis include fever, headache, stiff neck and neurological problems.

Treatment
This fungus is not particularly common in Europe, and can be treated using *amphotericin* and *flucytosine*, both of which may cause side-effects such as shivering and fevers. *Fluconazole* is a more recent option, but although it has fewer side-effects its efficacy in treating acute infection has not yet been proven.

Lymphoma, or cancer of the lymph nodes
Lymphoma can crop up in people with and without HIV, but in HIV-positive people is associated with the *Epstein Barr virus*. It can affect the brain primarily, but also may attack the skin, intestines and liver.

Treatment
Treatments include *radiotherapy* and *chemotherapy*.

Gastro-intestinal Infections

There are a range of infections in the stomach and intestines that can result from HIV-related immune deficiency.

Cryptosporidium
Cryptosporidium is a parasite that can be found in water supplies, and causes diarrhoea in cattle, children and adults with immune suppression. It inhabits the lining of the intestines, but it is still not

clear whether people with HIV develop cryptosporidiosis because they already have the infection and immune suppression allows it to flare up, or because they have become infected through tap water or through other people who have it.

Symptoms of cryptosporidiosis can be very serious in people with HIV, ranging from mild to excessive diarrhoea, acute abdominal pain and liver disease. The parasite seems to hinder the body's ability to absorb food, and the resultant diarrhoea can cause dehydration and malnutrition.

Treatment

There is still no specific cure for cryptosporidiosis. One of the problems with treating it is that its waxy outer coat prevents antibiotics from being effective, although zidovudine may help to improve immune deficiency and thus prevent it occurring or at least alleviate symptoms. However, some of the related symptoms, such as diarrhoea and stomach pain, can be treated with drugs like *imodium* and painkillers. Predigested food supplements and rehydration therapy can help prevent weight loss and dehydration through diarrhoea.

Cytomegalovirus, or CMV

CMV is a virus in the herpes virus family (see also *herpes zoster* and *herpes simplex*, above). It is transmitted through sex, saliva, blood, and from mother to child. A large proportion of the population are likely to have CMV infection, but it only seems to cause problems in people with immune suppression.

CMV can affect the eyes (see CMV *retinitis*, below), nervous system, intestines and, very rarely, the lungs. CMV colitis, however, tends to occur when the immune system has been severely damaged.

CMV colitis, or inflammation of the colon (the last part of the bowel), results in abdominal pain, diarrhoea, fever, and weight loss. It can also cause ulcers in the gullet.

Treatment

Treatments include *foscarnet* and *ganciclovir*; sometimes these are also administered as a preventive measure to prevent a recurrence of CMV colitis.

Candida albicans

This is a fungus which we all have. Generally our immune systems can control it, but factors such as illness, stress, poor diet, antibiotics or the contraceptive pill can allow it to thrive. In women, whether they are HIV positive or not, candida can cause thrush in the vagina (which can be treated with vaginal pessaries) and sometimes in the mouth. However, in women with HIV thrush is often longer-lasting and more severe (see *Women and HIV Illness*, below).

Candida infection can result in ulcers in the gullet; when it infects the small intestine it may finally lead to diarrhoea, malnutrition and weight loss.

Treatment

There are a number of treatments for it, including *fluconazole*. Eating live yoghourt may also be helpful for thrush generally, as the bacteria in yoghourt are thought to fight the fungus. It is a good idea to avoid sweet foods and starch if you have thrush, since the fungus feeds off sugary substances. Oral thrush is discussed further below, under *Oral Infections*.

Giardia lamblia and Salmonella

Bacterial and protozoal infections causing gastro-intestinal problems in people with HIV include *giardia lamblia* and types of *salmonella*. Bacterial infections in particular can affect people with healthy immune systems, but an infection like salmonella can spread into other parts of the body in people with immune weakness, and then lie dormant until reactivated by, say, a course of antibiotics.

Treatment

There is no specific treatment for salmonella or other bacterial infections; the best way to avoid them is by taking extra care about handling and preparing foods (see Chapter 7 for further information).

Mycobacterium tuberculosis

This can also affect the intestines as well as the lung, liver and lymph nodes. It generally occurs outside the lungs only in severely immune suppressed people.

Treatment

Treatment is the same as for TB in the lungs (see page 50).

Oral Infections

Oral and dental infections, such as abscesses, mouth ulcers and tooth decay, are common with HIV-related immune deficiency.

Candida albicans

This often causes inflammation of the lining of the mouth in people with HIV, forming white spots which should be quite easy to remove. There may also be sores at the corner of the mouth. (See also *Gastro-intestinal Infections*, above.)

Treatment

Candida albicans can be treated with live yoghourt, as suggested above, but other therapies for oral candidiasis include *amphotericin* lozenges, *nystatin* syrup and *fluconazole*.

Hairy oral leukoplakia

This condition only seems to affect people with immune suppression. It appears as white, warty patches on the side and bottom of the tongue and on the inner cheeks of people with HIV. It does not seem to cause pain or discomfort but, unlike oral candidiasis, cannot be scraped off. The condition is generally attributed to a viral infection, although it is unclear which virus (or viruses) may cause it.

Treatment

Hairy oral leukoplakia can be treated with *acyclovir*; it may also improve with *zidovudine* treatment. Some doctors regard the presence of hairy leukoplakia as an indication that more symptomatic HIV disease may develop.

Eye Infections

CMV Retinitis

CMV retinitis is an eye infection which can be particularly serious in people with HIV, and may cause total blindness if left untreated. It occurs when the retina of the eye (the 'screen' at the back of the eye on which images are formed) is damaged by CMV infection (see *cytomegalovirus*, above). Symptoms of this may be the perception of flashing lights, and partial blind spots.

Treatment

Early treatment with drugs like *ganciclovir* can be very effective in reversing CMV retinitis, although this may lead to anaemia, as ganciclovir affects the bone marrow. *Foscarnet* is an unlicensed drug in the UK at present, but has been shown to be almost as helpful as ganciclovir in treating CMV retinitis, and it may be possible to get the drug as a participant in a clinical trial (see Chapter 7).

Treatment for CMV retinitis rarely clears the infection away completely. This means that maintenance therapy of the above drugs may be necessary to avoid the infection recurring.

Thrombocytopenia

Finally, people with HIV infection may experience a condition called *thrombocytopenia*, which causes patches of bruising on the skin and occasional internal bleeding. This is caused by a decrease in the number of blood platelets, sometimes as a result of treatments for other HIV-related conditions. Such treatments may allow the blood cells of the immune system to get rid of platelets covered with HIV antibody - hence the patchy skin discolouring. Thrombocytopenia can also occur in people who have HIV but no symptoms of illness.

WOMEN AND HIV ILLNESS

Women with early HIV disease may experience recurrent and severe gynaecological infections. Vaginal candidiasis (thrush) and urinary tract infections such as cystitis, and genital warts, which are linked to disorders of the cervix such as inflammation and cancer, are more common among women with HIV infection. (It is notable that the cervix may also play a significant part in women's vulnerability to HIV infection through unsafe penetrative sex. The cervix responds to hormonal changes during a woman's menstrual cycle, and at certain times allows sperm into the uterus in order for pregnancy to occur, which may put women at particular risk of HIV infection.)

Other sexually transmitted diseases such as *chlamydia* (which can lead to pelvic inflammatory disease, or PID) may also be more prevalent, and generally produce no symptoms in women for several months before more serious disease may develop. HIV-related infections that women and men share include PCP, CMV, toxoplasmosis and oral thrush (see above). According to US studies, women are unlikely to develop HIV-related KS, which is most prevalent among gay men with HIV disease.

Although HIV infection is increasing rapidly among women world-wide, awareness of women's experience of HIV infection and their related medical and social needs remains limited. A key reason for this is that early on in the epidemic, gay men made up the vast majority of people with HIV in the UK (as elsewhere in western

Europe and in the US), and therefore information, support and counselling services for HIV-positive people were usually established with a male clientele in mind. In many cases, women with HIV have had to make do with such services, whether or not they were appropriate. Agencies providing care and support specifically for women with or concerned about HIV have only been established comparatively recently.

The attention paid to the health needs of women with HIV is affected by social and economic factors. In parts of the developing world, where resources for health care may be strictly limited, neither men nor women with HIV are likely to receive the medical attention and drug treatments available in richer countries.

However, the attention given to women's health needs may also be determined by the degree of social status they are accorded generally. Societies that view women primarily as care-givers and providers of support to others may not necessarily view them as equally worthy of care and support themselves. Women may decline to 'make demands' upon existing health services for practical reasons such as the burden of caring for young children or elderly family members. They may also be afraid that their symptoms will not be taken seriously, or may simply regard their own health needs as of little significance. A study of men and women with HIV in New York State found that the women put up with an average of 60 weeks of illness before asking for medical care; men sought medical help after an average of 24 weeks.

This reluctance or inability to put their own health needs first may have a serious effect on women's survival times with HIV. Research indicates that world-wide, men with HIV live longer than women with HIV. This cannot be explained by biological differences between the sexes. It is much more likely to be the result of delay in reaching medical services, coupled with a lack of recognition of women's HIV symptoms on the part of medical practitioners.

Women with HIV disease may be misdiagnosed or underdiagnosed for several reasons. Symptoms of HIV illness are, in many cases, common infections in HIV-negative women. Doctors may not automatically associate them with HIV infection, although the symptoms may be more severe and recurrent in HIV-positive women. Symptoms of HIV illness shared by men and women may also be interpreted differently by doctors. For example, substantial (and unintentional) weight loss is treated seriously in men with HIV, but may not necessarily be in women with HIV because western societies may view weight loss in women generally as a desirable goal.

All this means that the number of women with HIV is likely to be under-recorded. Until health carers have a clearer idea of women's experience of HIV illness, HIV-positive women may die of related infections before receiving an AIDS diagnosis. Consequently, they will not appear in the international AIDS statistics collated by the World Health Organization.

CHILDREN AND HIV ILLNESS

If you are caring for a child with HIV infection, the following section and the information given in Chapters 4 and 8 may be helpful. However, it is also very important to seek further advice and help from experienced health and social workers.

As for women, information about children's experience of HIV infection is limited. Children can become infected through contaminated blood supplies, like adults, or before birth if the mother is HIV positive. (HIV-positive women may also infect babies through breastfeeding, though there are still few recorded cases of this.)

Children infected by contaminated blood can be diagnosed through use of the HIV antibody test. However, one of the difficulties in diagnosing HIV infection in babies born to HIV-positive mothers is that all babies inherit their mothers' antibodies. The baby of a woman with HIV would therefore automatically test positive for HIV antibodies, because he or she would have received the mother's antibodies before birth. Babies lose maternal antibodies at around 18 months, so it is necessary to wait until then before the HIV antibody test can give an accurate result. By then, an HIV-positive baby is likely to have developed his or her own antibodies to HIV infection.

Currently, methods of HIV detection other than conventional antibody tests are being developed, but they are expensive and not yet ready for widespread use. In their absence, it may not be until a baby develops HIV illness that carers may realise that he or she has the virus. In some cases, it may also be the first indication to the baby's mother that she has HIV infection. As a baby's immune system is less developed than that of an adult, some HIV-positive babies become ill quickly. There is therefore little time for doctors to provide appropriate anti-viral treatments or preventive medicine to keep serious illness at bay.

Although there is still no 100 per cent effective therapy available to prevent or treat HIV illness, drug treatments have advanced considerably since the HIV epidemic began. As they continue to do so, it will become increasingly important for HIV to be detected early in babies and young children.

HIV illness in children may be indicated in the form of repeated bacterial infections (such as cytomegalovirus or thrush – see above), skin infections, lasting diarrhoea and stunted growth. Sometimes HIV-positive children may show delay in achieving developmental 'milestones', such as learning to walk and talk. As time goes on, they may become increasingly unable to perform tasks associated with healthy development in HIV-negative children of the same age. While such symptoms are not specific to HIV infection, they are important indicators in situations where the mother is known to be HIV positive.

Lung disease is common in children with HIV illness. *Lymphoid interstitital pneumonitis* (LIP) is a condition which has symptoms similar to PCP and involves the lungs filling up with lymphocytes. It is most common in children with HIV infection, but occurs occasionally in adults. LIP is characterised by swollen lymph glands, a fever, breathing problems and a dry, unproductive cough. Although it may be treated with steroids, it generally results in lasting damage to the lungs. Less commonly, HIV-positive children may develop PCP (see above).

Treatments for HIV illness in children include infusions of *gammaglobulin* for bacterial infections, *fluconazole* for oral thrush and *pentamidine* or *co-trimoxazole* for PCP. Research into the usefulness and safety of zidovudine in preventing or delaying the development of HIV illness in children continues. The fact that it is a toxic drug with severe side-effects may limit its potential as an effective treatment for HIV-positive children. However, early reports suggest that it may be helpful in dealing with HIV-related neurological illness in children such as encephalopathy (see above).

It is difficult to give hard and fast guidelines about children's survival times with HIV, since far more research into this area is needed. However, while factors such as access to health care services and appropriate drug therapies must be taken into account, a child with HIV is generally likely to fall ill more quickly and survive for a shorter period of time with HIV disease than will an adult.

Studies of infection in children born to HIV-positive mothers suggest that two broad patterns of disease may be distinguished. Children may develop symptoms of HIV illness within months after birth, or they may stay asymptomatic for a matter of years, in which case they are also likely to live longer with HIV illness.

Global estimates about the development of HIV infection in children appear relatively pessimistic; this is because they take into account the vast proportion of infected children living in countries where appropriate medical attention and treatment may not be available. The World Health Organization considers that 25 per cent of children infected by HIV-positive mothers may be diagnosed with AIDS before they are one year old; 45 per cent before they are two; 60 per cent before they are three and 80 per cent before they are four years of age.

Proper care for someone with HIV illness is not just a question of appropriate medical treatment; it is also about provision of information, practical help, advice and support. The psychological effects of learning to live with HIV infection or AIDS can be enormous, including severe shock, anger, depression and anxiety. Chapters 6 and 7 look at these issues in more detail.

VACCINE RESEARCH AND DRUG TREATMENTS

Vaccines

Scientists attempting to develop a vaccine against HIV infection are faced with a very tall order. The virus invades, and may ultimately destroy, exactly those cells which are designed to inactivate infectious agents. Also, there is still no absolute scientific proof that it is possible for the human body to develop immunity to HIV infection.

Normally, infection with a micro-organism causes the body to manufacture antibodies and other special cells to get rid of the invading agent. Providing that the person recovers from the illness, the next time that the body is infected by the same organism, cells within the immune system are able to recognise the infection and deal with it more rapidly, before disease can develop. The body thus has an in-built 'memory' of previous infections, and develops immunity to them. It is this process that vaccines attempt to copy, without the person concerned having to become ill to begin with.

However, with HIV infection, the antibodies that are produced by the body are ineffective in getting rid of the virus. People with HIV do not appear to get rid of the virus nor to develop an immunity to further infection. Instead the virus seems to stay with them for the rest of their lives.

There are other reasons why producing a vaccine against HIV will be difficult. Vaccines for other infections are often tested on animals which have been injected with the organism causing disease. If the vaccine works on the animal, then it is considered likely to work on people also. HIV, however, only seems to affect humans, and although it is possible to infect chimpanzees with the virus, none have so far developed disease. Apart from the scientific uncertainty surrounding this approach, it is morally dubious: chimpanzees are highly intelligent, and are in danger of extinction. They are also expensive, costing up to £25,000 each.

Vaccine research for other infections has relied on identifying the part of a micro-organism which stimulates the immune system to respond, then building this part of the agent into a vaccine which will prompt an immune response without causing illness. With HIV, it is unclear which part of the virus is responsible for provoking the immune system's response. Even if this were apparent, we cannot be certain that a vaccine incorporating this part of the virus would work, since all the evidence suggests that the body's immune response to HIV infection does not seem to get rid of the virus. A further difficulty is that HIV, like many other viruses, mutates rapidly. Even within a single individual, the strain of HIV may change over time. The fact that HIV is able to change in this way makes it very hard for the immune system to remember and respond to it.

Despite these drawbacks research has continued, and scientists at the sixth international AIDS conference in June 1990 were reported to be 'cautiously optimistic' that an effective vaccine could be developed against HIV infection by the year 2000. Current studies include work with animals that are infected with similar, if not identical, viruses. Cats and monkeys, for example, are prone to infections produced by retroviruses which may lead to symptoms of immune weakness. The *Simian Immunodeficiency Virus* (SIV) is related to HIV, and can lead to immune deficiency in some types of monkey, such as the macaque. Researchers hope that by looking at the way retroviruses affect the immune system of other animals, they may develop vaccines against these and use the same technology to produce one which can protect against HIV infection in humans.

A number of research projects into HIV vaccines have looked at using other live viruses, such as *vaccinia* (the virus that causes smallpox) and inserting genes from HIV into them. The idea behind this is that it is important for viral proteins to be presented to the immune system in a specific way, as part of another virus for example, in order to stimulate an effective response. However, there are distinct disadvantages to this approach. Injecting people whose immune systems are already stressed by HIV with another live virus could lead to disease; by straining the body's defences further, it could result in the development of HIV illness.

One way of getting around these problems is by developing a synthetic virus. British Biotechnology, a research company based in Oxford, has managed to do this in collaboration with a team of British researchers. The 'fake virus' consists of proteins from yeast cells combined with parts of the envelope protein of HIV. The yeast particles carry the HIV protein on their surface and, it is hoped, will stimulate the human immune system to produce antibodies to the virus. The vaccine is called *p24-VLP* (virus-like particle) because the HIV protein it uses is called p24. Its major advantage is that it is not infectious and so cannot cause disease. The vaccine has been tested on animals and was successful in producing antibodies against HIV. It is now being tested on human volunteers in London who do not already have HIV and are in a good state of health.

Vaccines are generally viewed as a form of protection for people who have not already encountered a particular micro-organism. In theory, they may also be successful in preventing the onset of disease in people who are already infected. After all, if it is possible to produce effective antibodies to a virus to prevent infection in the first place, the same antibodies may be useful in stopping the infection causing disease. In 1987, research began into the possibility of producing a vaccine to delay the development of AIDS in people who are HIV positive.

Jonas Salk, the American scientist who developed the anti-polio vaccine in 1954, has collaborated with the Immune Response Corporation in California to produce a vaccine made from quantities of whole, irradiated virus. The radiation process inactivates HIV so that it can no longer infect cells, and the vaccine is then given to volunteers who already have the virus, but no symptoms of infection. Trials have been designed to see whether the HIV-positive volunteers in the group who receive the treatment will take longer to develop AIDS than those who receive a placebo. By 1989, Salk claimed that the medical condition of 17 out of 19 people who were ill with HIV disease had 'stabilised' after receiving his vaccine; in early 1990 he stated that the vaccine trials would expand to involve a larger number of people.

The participation of people who are already HIV positive is considered to circumvent ethical problems that would arise from giving a treatment containing viral genetic material (even if the virus has been inactivated through irradiation) to uninfected people. Even so, critics of Salk's approach state that active HIV might survive the irradiation process and thereby increase levels of infection in volunteers. For this reason, Salk has said that he will try the vaccine on himself, and expects to present the first results from the trials in 1992.

While some scientists suggest that an effective vaccine could be available by as early as 1995 or 1996, there are those who have doubts that a vaccine against HIV could ever be fully effective. Some of the reasons for this are discussed above, but another factor in the argument is that antibodies alone may never be adequate to provide immunity. Far less is known about the part played by other cells in the immune system than about antibodies, but it seems likely that HIV is transmitted between people not just by free virus, but also by cells infected with the virus. Researchers argue therefore that a vaccine which only stimulates the body to produce antibodies cannot work properly; specialised cells within the immune system may also need to be set into action.

Whether or not these researchers are right still remains to be seen. The development of an effective vaccine is, however, only half the story. Establishing ethical procedures for testing possible treatments raises another set of questions. New vaccines for other infections have generally been trialled on large groups of people thought to be at risk from the relevant infection. Researchers then look at whether those who received the vaccine were less prone to disease than those who did not. In many cases (such as for smallpox) people were not in a position to avoid infection, and so had little to lose from vaccination. This is not so with HIV infection.

Participants in trials for an HIV vaccine would need to be told the possible infection risks involved. At the same time, researchers would be ethically bound to provide education about staying safe from HIV. It would therefore automatically become more difficult to analyse the effectiveness of the vaccine treatment, because if participants practised safer behaviour there would be no infection for the vaccine to work against.

Discussion of trialling vaccines among people considered to be 'at high risk' of HIV ~ such as gay men or injecting drug users ~ focuses on the idea that as there is likely to be a greater exposure to infection in these groups, assessment of the vaccine's success against HIV would be easier to undertake. However, this in no way avoids the ethical dilemma of administering a potentially risky treatment to people who do not already have HIV. Similarly, there would still need to be an obligation for the participants involved to be thoroughly educated about avoiding infection.

Vaccine trials would also have to find a way of distinguishing between people who have developed antibodies to the virus in response to a vaccine and people who have produced antibodies anyway because they have HIV infection. This is problematic, because insurers are reluctant to provide cover for people with HIV, and therefore people vaccinated with HIV antibodies could find themselves in the same situation, that is, having to prove that they are not infected. This would be hard to do, considering that available tests for HIV measure the presence of antibodies to the virus, not HIV itself (see Chapter 6).

For these reasons, British researchers have called for internationally agreed guidelines on testing procedures for HIV vaccines. As yet, however, scientists are still in disagreement about relevant criteria for setting up fair and effective vaccine trials.

Drug Treatments for HIV Infection and Related Illness

Treatments which attempt to delay the action of HIV upon the immune system have to confront the fact that it is very hard to attack the virus without also damaging the cells into which it has entered. A second difficulty is that HIV is able to affect the brain directly, by hiding in the nervous system where it cannot be tackled by drugs circulating in the bloodstream. In order to cope with the illnesses that result from immune deficiency, and to delay or hinder the impact of HIV upon the body, three broad categories of drug have been developed: prophylactics, anti-retroviral drugs and immunorestoratives.

Prophylactics

There are drugs used to treat opportunistic infections. Where these have a preventive role they are called *prophylactics*. An example of such a drug is nebulised pentamidine for the prevention of PCP. Other examples are given under the relevant infection listed in the section above.

Anti-retroviral Drugs

There are *anti-retroviral drugs*, which work against HIV itself. These can take effect in a number of ways. Zidovudine is the only anti-retroviral drug licensed in Britain to deal with HIV at the time of writing. It works by blocking the reverse transcriptase enzyme inside HIV that allows the virus to reproduce itself inside the infected cell. Drugs that interrupt the reproductive process of the virus in this way are called *nucleoside analogues*.

People with HIV illness who are on zidovudine have reported benefits such as long periods of good health, increased T4 cell levels and a decline in the amount of HIV proteins detectable in their blood. There is little doubt that zidovudine has improved the quality of life for many people with HIV illness, but the drug is far from being a cure. It may slow the action of HIV in the body, but it cannot inactivate the virus permanently. Some people who stop taking zidovudine experience severe illness following a resultant burst of viral activity.

Zidovudine is also a toxic drug. It can result in severe side-effects, including anaemia, headaches, nausea, damage to the bone marrow and, in some cases, muscular wasting. Some of these problems may be avoided once an appropriate minimum effective dosage has been found for HIV-symptomatic people. Combining zidovudine with other anti-viral drugs such as dideoxyinosine, or DDI, and dideoxycytidine, or DDC (both are nucleoside analogues, like zidovudine) may also allow lower dosage levels and fewer side-effects. A trial called the Delta Trial was set up in mid-1991 to look at the efficacy and toxicity of combining AZT with either DDI or DDC. One third of the participants will receive AZT and DDI, one third AZT and DDC, and one third AZT and a placebo. Participants will be allocated their respective dosages at random.

It is still not clear how zidovudine will affect people with HIV illness in the longer term, as the drug has only been in use for a comparatively short time. One possible difficulty is that people taking zidovudine could develop an increasing resistance to it, so its use might have to be limited to short periods only. For symptomatic people with HIV who have become resistant to zidovudine, other anti-retroviral drugs such as DDI (see below) may be an effective replacement.

There is a continuing debate about the value of *asymptomatic* people with HIV taking zidovudine to prevent or delay future disease. Part of the problem lies in healthy people taking a drug known to have toxic side-effects; another issue is that of resistance. Some doctors and people with HIV feel that an asymptomatic person with HIV may have to take zidovudine for a long time (the asymptomatic period of infection may last for a number of years). This could enable resistance to the drug to develop, so that it would be ineffective if HIV illness occurred.

On the other hand, those in favour of asymptomatic people with HIV taking zidovudine argue that the drug may not necessarily cause resistance. They also argue that even if resistance does occur, there are other anti-retroviral therapies being developed to replace zidovudine. At the moment there are no easy answers to this question, as considerably more research is needed. A major trial of zidovudine for asymptomatic people with HIV began in October 1988 and is currently still under way in both British and French clinics.

A third area of uncertainty among researchers is the impact of zidovudine upon the health of women and children with HIV disease. Again, this is an area where a great deal more information is necessary. Setting appropriate dosage levels of zidovudine for women requires further research, and it is unclear whether the drug can be effectively used to treat children with the virus anyway (see *Children and HIV Illness*, above). The development of clinical drug trials which represent the needs of women and children with HIV, as well as men, is an issue discussed in more detail in Chapter 9.

DDI (see above) is an anti-retroviral drug closely related to zidovudine. It is considered to be less toxic than zidovudine, and does not cause bone marrow damage (which can lead to anaemia). It is not, however, without side-effects, which may include inflammation of the pancreas, abdominal pain and fever. Like zidovudine, DDI is not a cure. There is, however, a great deal of hope that the drug might go a long way towards improving the quality of life for people with HIV illness who can no longer take zidovudine.

A British trial of DDI was set up in May 1990, and is open to anyone with HIV who has taken zidovudine but has come off the drug because of its side-effects. Participants on the trial are able to continue taking other drugs, and can opt to receive no treatment (a placebo) if they wish, or to receive DDI, which will be given at two different dosage levels.

This ability to choose between treatment or a placebo is important; in previous drug trials people with HIV may have wanted a particular treatment but had no information or choice about whether they were allocated a placebo or the relevant drug. This lack of choice has been labelled 'placebo roulette' by AIDS activists; the argument behind it is that it prevents 'psychological' factors from muddying the trial results. (In other words, it would be hard to know whether any changes in health in trial participants resulted from the action of the drug or from participants' possible relief or anxiety about receiving it.)

If a drug shows signs of being effective against HIV, there are obvious ethical concerns in organising trials where people have no say in whether or not they receive it. At the same time, drugs such as DDI are toxic. Until there is clearer information about their effect on the body, some trial participants may want to have the option of receiving a placebo.

Another approach to preventing HIV from infecting the cells of the immune system is by stopping it from locking on to the cell membrane. The CD4 molecule on the surface of cells is the site to which the virus attaches itself; it may therefore be useful to create a synthetic CD4 molecule which would act as a sort of 'decoy' to the virus. In other words, the genetically engineered CD4 would be a free-floating substance in the blood which would 'mop up' HIV, preventing it from latching on to the CD4 molecule on T-cells. This approach has worked in the test tube, and trials are underway to see how safe and effective it is in people. One current drawback is that artificial CD4 of this sort would have to be administered by injection or drip.

Other types of anti-retroviral drug include *anti-oxidants*. Anti-oxidants aim to prevent oxidants from activating HIV. An example which is used in HIV treatment is vitamin C. Vitamin C has not yet been formally trialled and may cause diarrhoea and kidney problems.

Immunotherapy is a method of boosting the immune system's response to HIV. This is distinct from *immunorestoratives* (see below), which aim to bolster the immune system generally, not just in response to HIV. Immunotherapy works by injecting inactivated HIV or HIV antibodies into a person with the virus, in the hope that this will strengthen the immune system and prompt it to react more powerfully against the virus. Another technique, called *adoptive immunotherapy*, consists of injecting a person with cells that have been 'trained' to respond well to HIV. Studies of immunotherapy techniques are still underway, with some promising results to date.

Immunorestoratives

Alpha interferon is the only immunorestorative drug licensed in the UK at present (interferons are chemicals which the body produces to respond to infection or tumours). Alpha interferon has been found to have the dual benefit of slowing HIV activity and provoking lymphocytes in the immune system to attack cancerous or infected cells. It is being trialled widely on its own and with other drug therapies, but uncertainty remains about its effects. While it has proved to be very effective in the treatment of Kaposi's sarcoma, it can cause a drop in the levels of T4 cells in a person with HIV. In boosting the immune system, it is possible that alpha interferon may also boost the activity of HIV.

PREVENTING HIV THROUGH BEHAVIOUR CHANGE

At present, despite the enormous amount that has been learned about HIV and AIDS, there is still no effective vaccine to prevent HIV infection. Similarly, there is no treatment that can be said to be a 'cure', although, as shown above, drugs have been developed with increasing success to deal both with the direct impact of HIV upon the body's immune system and with the resulting illnesses.

The only means of HIV prevention currently available to us is staying safe from infection by making appropriate behaviour changes. Chapter 3 looks at how HIV is and is not transmitted. Chapters 4 and 5 give basic information and guidelines for safer behaviour.

3

HIV TRANSMISSION

FACTS AND FICTION

At 'Hysteria', a benefit evening in 1989 to raise money for the Terrence Higgins Trust, actor and comedian Stephen Fry told a joke about AIDS, which went like this.

A man goes into a pub and orders a pint of beer in a tankard glass. He pays for the beer, takes it and sits down. To the barman's surprise, he begins drinking the beer from the tankard just above where the handle joins the glass, so that his chin keeps knocking the handle, and beer slops all over his shirt. He finishes the pint in this way, with most of the beer going over his clothing and very little into his mouth. When he goes up to the bar to take the glass back, the barman decides to bring the matter up.

'Excuse me, mate,' he says, 'but I couldn't help noticing . . . why did you drink your pint with your mouth just above the handle of the glass? Your shirt's soaked with beer.'

'Well – it's this AIDS scare, you see,' replies the man. 'I reckon if you drink from the glass just above the handle, no one else will have been drinking from that bit, so I won't get AIDS'.

A few days later, another man comes in to the pub, and orders a pint of beer in a tankard glass. He sits down, and, exactly like the first man, begins drinking from the glass just above the handle. His chin knocks the handle and beer slops all over his clothes.

When he takes the empty glass back to the bar, the barman says 'I saw you drinking your beer from the glass just above the handle. Is that because you're worried about AIDS?'

The man looks at him. 'No,' he says, 'actually I already have the virus. I know you can't pass it on through saliva and so on, but I was just being extra specially careful.'

A QUESTION OF RISK

The subject of HIV infection presents us all with a series of questions about the way we live and the risks we are prepared to

73

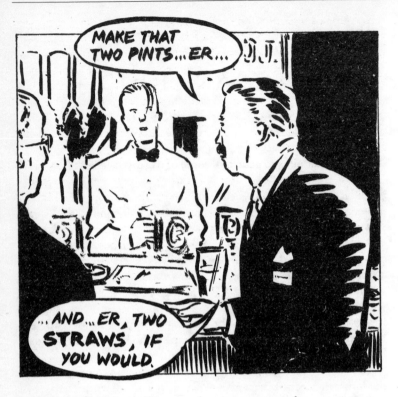

take in our daily lives. We may choose to ignore the questions, or we may choose to answer them. Whatever decision we make is likely to involve some sort of assessment of what risk means for us.

We take risks all the time, often without realising or thinking about it. Crossing the road, smoking a cigarette, or riding a bicycle in heavy traffic are all risks that may be commonplace and meaningless for some people; what seems an acceptable risk for some of us may be unthinkable for others. Our perception of personal risk may depend on factors such as past experience, what people tell us, or our own feelings of threat or excitement at the time. There is little doubt that a life completely free of risk-taking would be a pretty boring one, but the fact that we have no common yardstick for measuring what we might consider day-to-day risks does not make it easier for us to understand and confront the risk of serious illness or loss of life.

We are not helped in our assessment of risk by the way we sometimes receive information about HIV and AIDS. For many people, newspapers, television and gossip are the key providers, which presents problems because the stories we read or hear often conflict with each other. That which appears to be established fact one day is disputed elsewhere the next. This is confusing, and may make us panic about the risks HIV presents to us and how much control we have over our lives. Alternatively, we may get bored and 'switch off', allocating the possible threat of HIV to the safe compartment of 'someone else's risk, not mine'. The trouble is that the price of denying the risk of infection is considerably higher than most of us may want to acknowledge.

This chapter aims to get rid of some of the myths about how HIV is, and is *not*, transmitted. It is also meant to reassure. There is still no proven cure for HIV, nor an effective vaccine to prevent infection in people who do not have the virus or delay illness in those who do. However, it *is* possible to stay safe from infection: HIV is only passed between people in very limited ways, whereas the list of day-to-day activities that carry no risk of passing on the virus is enormous.

HIV AND BODY FLUIDS

HIV has been identified in laboratory research in the following body fluids of an HIV-positive person: blood, breastmilk, urine, faeces, semen, saliva, vaginal secretions, rectal secretions and the fluid around the brain.

However, the fact that HIV is present in these body fluids does not mean that contact with them will necessarily transmit the virus. In fact, it appears that the only body fluids capable of passing on HIV are infected blood, semen and vaginal secretions, and possibly breastmilk. One reason for this is probably that in the other body fluids (urine, faeces, saliva, rectal secretions and the fluid around the brain) there is not enough HIV present to cause effective transmission.

Even in a situation where a person is exposed to HIV infection, it is by no means certain that he or she will become infected, as indicated by studies of couples where one partner has HIV and regular unsafe sex has taken place. In some cases, HIV transmission has occurred between sexual partners after just one occasion of unsafe sex; in others, it has not occurred at all, even after frequent unsafe sexual activity.

One very important factor in the likelihood of HIV transmission occurring is the *amount* of virus to which a person is exposed. The amount of virus in an HIV-positive person increases in the few months following the date of infection, as well as at the point of becoming ill with HIV disease (Chapter 2 explains this in greater detail). This means that at those times he or she may be more infectious to other people. It does *not* mean that the ways in which HIV can be transmitted to other people are any different.

The next two sections give information about how HIV is and is not transmitted. More detailed guidance on staying safe and protecting other people from HIV is given in Chapters 4 and 5, which look in depth at the main routes of HIV transmission. The most important starting point for reading what follows is to remember that no one can tell from appearances or guesswork who has HIV infection and who has not. Similarly, if you have been in situations identified below as risky for HIV transmission, it is impossible to be certain whether you have HIV or not without taking the HIV antibody test (this is explained fully in Chapter 6).

Facing these facts means coping with a considerable degree of uncertainty. However, false assumptions about who is and who is not likely to have HIV infection are highly dangerous. For that reason, the best advice is always to practise safer behaviour: that is one thing of which we can be absolutely certain.

HOW HIV IS TRANSMITTED

For HIV to be passed on, the virus has to be able to enter another person's bloodstream in sufficient quantity to cause infection. It is not transmitted through the air, so can only be effectively passed on when infected blood, semen, vaginal secretions or breastmilk get into another person's body. As healthy skin is a very good barrier to infection, there are only a few ways in which this can happen.

Blood-to-blood Contact

The first way is blood-to-blood contact, or, in other words, situations where infected blood (or blood products) get into the body of another person. There are a number of ways in which this can happen. If a person is given a blood transfusion and the blood is infected, the chances of HIV transmission are high because a large amount of the virus is able to go straight into the bloodstream. In Britain, and in other places where all blood donations have been tested for HIV antibodies since 1985, the chances of getting HIV through a blood transfusion are now negligible. Similarly, blood products are treated in order to inactivate HIV in the UK. Chapter 4 gives more detailed information about this.

Accidents involving contact with infected blood in occupational settings, such as health care work, are also a route of HIV transmission, although to date there are very few reported cases of this, and the risk seems to be extremely low. Data compiled and reported in April 1990 by the Communicable Disease Surveillance Centre (CDSC) in London indicated only 33 documented cases internationally of health workers becoming HIV positive after accidents with infected blood.

Needlestick injuries (jabbing yourself with a needle accidentally) or other accidents with sharp instruments (such as scissors) are a reasonably common occurrence for health care workers. There is a risk of HIV transmission if a sharp instrument with HIV-infected blood on it punctures a person's skin, because the infected blood can thereby enter his or her body. However the risk remains very low, both because of the minute quantity of infected blood involved and because wounds on the body bleed *outwards* in order to stay clean (so that it is relatively difficult for HIV to be absorbed). The transmission rate is thought to be around 1 in 200 for each accidental exposure to HIV infected blood, or less than 0.5 per cent.

Skin-piercing instruments may put you at risk of HIV transmission if they are shared and inadequately sterilised. It is therefore a good idea to check standards of hygiene if you are having a tattoo done, getting your ears or nose pierced, visiting an acupuncturist or receiving medical injections of any sort. Many practitioners, particularly medical personnel, are now very well informed and careful about HIV risks that result from inadequate sterilisation of equipment. If you are worried, asking your practitioner about sterilisation methods should serve to reassure you. If it does not, you could think of going elsewhere.

HIV transmission might also occur accidentally if blood from a person with HIV is able to get into the body through broken skin or through the surfaces of the eyes and mouth, although again there are very few recorded cases of this happening. If you are in a situation where you have to deal with another person's blood, remember to keep wounds on your skin covered and to wear disposable gloves to mop up blood spillages. Further information about protecting yourself from accidental infection in the workplace and other settings is given in Chapter 4.

Finally, sharing equipment ('works') to inject drugs has become an increasingly common route of HIV transmission. In the process of injecting a drug, blood often enters both the needle and the syringe. If the syringe and needle are then shared with someone else, that person will inject any blood that has stayed behind in the equipment, along with the drug. Sharing mixing equipment, such as the bowl and spoon used to dissolve the drug with water, may also be risky, because traces of blood may remain on it and be injected with the drug.

One of the reasons why sharing equipment to inject drugs is such an effective method of HIV transmission is because a substantial amount of infected blood may be injected directly into another person's body. Keeping a clean supply of equipment which is not shared with anyone is one way to avoid HIV infection in injecting drug use. Another is to sterilise injecting equipment (see Chapter 4 for more information about safer injecting drug use).

Sexual Transmission

Infected vaginal fluids, semen and blood can transmit HIV if they are able to get into another person's body during sexual intercourse. This is now the most common route of HIV transmission world-wide, and applies to all sexually active people, whether we see ourselves as gay, bisexual or heterosexual. HIV cannot distinguish sexual identity. Who you are does not matter; it is what you do that counts.

Penetrative sex ('screwing' or 'fucking'), where a man puts his penis into his partner's vagina or anus, is unsafe. Infected semen can be absorbed into the partner's bloodstream through the walls of the vagina and/or anus. Similarly, infected vaginal fluid, or blood from the vagina or anus, may be absorbed through the skin of the penis and through the lining of the urethra (the narrow tube inside the penis through which a man urinates). HIV also exists in the clear fluid that sometimes comes from the penis before a man has ejaculated, known as 'pre-ejaculate' or 'pre-come'. This means that withdrawal of the penis before orgasm does not prevent HIV infection to the person who is receiving the penis. Similarly, it does not protect the man whose penis it is from being infected through vaginal fluid or blood from his partner's body.

One effective way of reducing the risks of HIV transmission during penetrative sex is by using a condom. Far from being a fiddly and embarrassing piece of latex that is sold as 'something for the weekend' from downmarket men's hairdressers, clever publicity has attempted to transform the condom into a sexy fashion accessory for the streetwise man and woman. A poster campaign launched in 1991 by the Terrence Higgins Trust featured an androgynous cartoon character sporting a large pink condom as a halo, with the caption 'Be Good in Bed'. In the United States, some brands of condom are said to have been marketed in different sizes to meet all needs: 'large', 'extra large', and 'liar'.

While it is still uncertain whether such marketing techniques will be successful in encouraging men to buy and use condoms, what is clear is that condoms make penetrative sex safer. Infected semen is held inside the condom, so it cannot make contact with the vagina or anus, and infected blood or vaginal fluid cannot make contact with the penis, because the condom is in the way.

The use of lubricants during penetration may also play an important role in keeping sex safer. This is particularly true for anal sex, since the anus tends to be drier and tighter than the vagina and therefore possibly more vulnerable to friction and bleeding. Chapter 5 has more information on condoms and lubricants.

During unsafe penetrative sex between men and women or between two men, it is the 'receptive' person (the one who is being penetrated by his or her partner's penis) who is more at risk than is the 'active' person (the man whose penis is penetrating his partner). This means two things. The first is that women are generally more at risk of HIV infection through unsafe penetrative sex with men than vice versa. Secondly, men who have sex with men are considered to be more at risk of HIV through unsafe penetrative sex if they are 'receptive' rather than 'active' partners.

One reason for this may be that quantities of infected semen can remain behind for some time in the vagina or anus, giving HIV more opportunity to be absorbed into the bloodstream. Infected vaginal fluid or blood from the receptive person may not be in contact with the penis for long, so HIV transmission is considered to be less risky for the 'active' person. Another probable factor is that the skin inside the vagina and anus may be damaged more easily during penetrative sex than is the skin of the penis, allowing infected semen an opportunity to enter the bloodstream of the receptive partner.

There is, however, another reason why women are considered to be more at risk of HIV infection than are men as a result of unsafe penetrative sex. Erosion of the cervix, which has a range of causes, may allow infected semen an increased chance of entering a woman's bloodstream during sex. Long-term studies of heterosexual couples where one person has HIV infection show that HIV-positive women have a 5 per cent to 15 per cent chance of passing the virus on to their male partner over a two- to three-year period through unsafe sex. According to the studies, the chance of men with HIV infecting their female partners through unsafe sex over the same period is twice as high, at between 10 per cent and 30 per cent.

Cuts or ulcers on or inside the genitals also make HIV transmission during penetrative sex more likely, because they provide points of entry for the virus. If the anus or vagina is inadequately lubricated, bruising and bleeding may occur during sex, and this may also increase the chances of HIV transmission. Any activity which damages the sensitive vaginal or anal walls and may lead to bleeding - such as inserting the fist into the vagina or anus, or scratches caused by long fingernails or jewellery - is likely to increase the risk of HIV infection. It puts the 'receptive' person more at risk because tears in the vaginal or anal skin may allow infected semen to enter the bloodstream; it may also put the penetrating partner at risk because of possible contact with infected blood.

In contrast, sex between women is considered to be fairly safe. Substantial amounts of infected vaginal fluid or blood are unlikely to be able to pass easily from a woman's body into that of her female sexual partner. As no penis is involved, infected semen cannot enter a partner's body and be absorbed into the bloodstream. Even so, women who have sex with women cannot rule out the risks of HIV transmission through sex entirely, and may need to be aware of other routes of infection. There may, for example, be a risk of HIV infection through contact with infected blood and blood products, through sharing equipment to inject drugs, and through sex with men.

At the time of writing, there is only one recorded case globally of a woman infected with HIV through sex with a female partner. At the same time, international studies of HIV transmission between women who have sex with women have been extremely limited. Whilst sex between women is undoubtedly safer than penetration involving a penis, the absence of evidence that women are at risk of HIV infection through sex with each other may be partly due to the acute lack of research in this area as well as to the type of sexual activity involved.

It is, however, heterosexual men and women who make up the vast majority of people with HIV and AIDS on a global basis, as reports from the World Health Organization indicate. In Britain, the number of heterosexual men and women with AIDS was reported by the Department of Health in October 1990 to have almost doubled during the course of the year: the rate of increase was 95 per cent, higher than in any other group. Although in Britain heterosexuals still form a minority of people with HIV and AIDS according to Government statistics, it is possible that by 1994 (in the absence of a vaccine against HIV infection or substantial changes in sexual behaviour) they could make up a significant majority.

While it is clear that having unsafe sex poses risks of HIV infection for everyone, people who seek to know the exact statistical risk of HIV infection in any specific sexual activity will always be disappointed, because such an assessment is an impossibility. A person who is exposed to infection cannot know how much virus has got into his or her body.

However, there is a basic rule to bear in mind, which can help to assess the safety of any given sexual activity. Sex which involves blood, semen or vaginal fluids getting *on* to a partner's body is safer; sex which allows them to get *in* to a partner's body is unsafe. Healthy, unbroken skin on the body is a barrier to HIV, as it is to other viruses.

This means that there is a wide range of sexual activities which remove or lessen the risk of HIV transmission. Safer sex need not be just about using condoms: it can offer some enormously exciting and sensual possibilities that have nothing to do with penetration (see Chapter 5).

Mother-to-baby Transmission

HIV can be transmitted from a pregnant woman with the virus to her baby both before birth, because the virus is able to cross the placenta and reach the foetus, and possibly after birth, through infected breastmilk.

It is by no means certain that a pregnant woman with HIV will pass the virus to her baby. Early studies, which involved women who were already ill with HIV-related disease, suggested that the chances of passing HIV on in this way were about 1 in 2, or 50 per cent.

Further research, however, has shown that this is a pessimistic estimate. For women who have HIV but no symptoms of illness, the rate of transmission could be as low as 20 per cent, according to findings from an ongoing major international study of children born to women with HIV in Europe. Initial fears that pregnancy might hasten the onset of illness in women with HIV (because it places a strain on the immune system) also appear to be unfounded. Chapter 4 gives further information on all aspects of HIV transmission and pregnancy.

HOW HIV IS *NOT* TRANSMITTED

There are many, many ways in which HIV is not transmitted. In fact, HIV is not a virus which can be transmitted through day-to-day social contact at all. It is not spread through the air or through saliva, through touch or proximity to a person with HIV. This means that some extremely pleasurable activities – talking, eating, drinking, and other aspects of social contact – are all safe as far as HIV infection is concerned. It also means that sex, one of the most popular of all pursuits, can be safe if we explore ways of giving ourselves pleasure without exchanging infected blood or genital fluids.

Since this is so, there is no reason for people with HIV to avoid social or sexual contact, or for other people to keep their distance. Myths about HIV as a socially transmittable virus have caused needless fears of infection and created hostility towards people living with HIV. The following are just some of the activities that people have worried about and which do *not* transmit HIV.

Breathing

HIV is not passed on by breathing air near a person with the virus. It is not transmitted in the water vapour created when we breathe, so sitting or standing close to a person with HIV is not a risk.

Saliva

Although HIV has been found in saliva, it is in such tiny amounts that transmission through saliva would not be possible. (Some scientists also suggest that there is a substance in saliva which inactivates the virus.) This means that activities such as sharing cups, cigarettes, cutlery and crockery – in fact any occasion where we may have contact with other people's saliva – are safe. It also means that kissing is safe, despite regularly-voiced fears about this.

Worries about HIV transmission occurring through bites can also be laid to rest. An American study published in late 1990 of 39 people who had been bitten (so that their skin was broken) by a person with HIV revealed that none of the 39 had become infected as a result. Anecdotal reports among family members bitten by a child with HIV, or carers bitten by infected hospital patients also show that biting is not an effective route of HIV transmission.

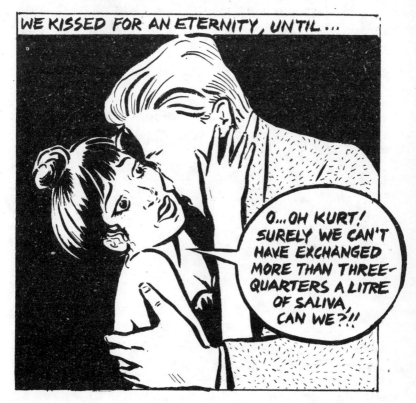

Physical Contact

Healthy, unbroken skin is an excellent barrier to HIV. As explained above, infected blood, semen and vaginal fluids need to get into a person's bloodstream before HIV transmission can occur, and the ways in which they can do this are limited. Touching, tickling, stroking, cuddling, hugging, massage, and shaking or holding hands are all safe, as is any contact with another person's unbroken skin. Keeping cuts covered up is a good hygienic precaution as well as an effective HIV prevention measure. Even so, there are *no* recorded cases anywhere in the world of HIV infection through social contact.

Workplace Contact

Some of the worst cases of unnecessary discrimination against people with HIV and AIDS have occurred in workplace settings.

As is made clear above, social contact provides no risk of HIV transmission. Sharing telephones, computers, cloakrooms, office space or factory space, canteen facilities and so on poses no risk. However, if you have (or plan to have) a sexual relationship with a colleague, you should read Chapter 5 on safer sex.

Clothes, Towels, and Bedlinen

HIV is fragile outside the body, and heat renders it inactive. The hot cycle in a washing machine is quite enough to deal with spilled body fluids such as blood or semen on clothes or linen, and so is ordinary household detergent or washing powder.

There is no risk of HIV transmission from sharing, or general contact with, the clothes and bedlinen of a person with HIV. It is unlikely that one would choose to wear someone else's clothes if they had spilled body fluid such as fresh blood on them, but it is sensible to avoid this.

Toilets and Washing Facilities

Toilet seats have always loomed large in HIV transmission mythology. In fact, ever since sit-down toilets were invented they have been blamed for a large number of unpleasant infections, including gonorrhoea, syphilis and now, HIV. Despite this, toilet seats have never and could never pass on HIV. It is therefore wise to ignore clever marketing for new toilet seat wipes, or special disinfectants designed to 'kill the virus'. They are often expensive, always unnecessary, and may lead you to think that HIV is far more easily transmitted than is the case. Similarly, there is no risk of HIV infection through sharing baths, showers, or wash-basins with a person who has the virus.

Sanitary Towels and Tampons

HIV has never been shown to be transmitted by disposal of used sanitary towels and tampons, for the very good reason that the person who is menstruating is generally the person who is doing the disposing. If you are caring for someone who is unable to take care of her own menstrual needs, the risks are still extremely low. Keep open cuts on your hands covered so there is no possibility of blood-to-blood contact, or wear disposable latex gloves. Used tampons can generally be flushed down the toilet, and used sanitary towels can most safely be disposed of in an incinerator, or wrapped in a plastic bag and thrown away.

Insects

Mosquitoes, bedbugs, headlice, fleas, and any other insects are all incapable of transmitting HIV. Insects which bite take such tiny amounts of blood that viral transmission just cannot take place. In theory, if hundreds of bedbugs (for example) bit a person with HIV at the same time and then rushed off together to bite another person, the risk might be slightly increased. However, bedbugs are extremely unlikely to behave in such an organised fashion outside the more fanciful realms of science fiction.

First Aid

Following standard hygienic precautions, such as wearing disposable gloves to deal with blood spillages and covering wounds on the body with bandages or sticking plaster, are quite adequate to prevent HIV

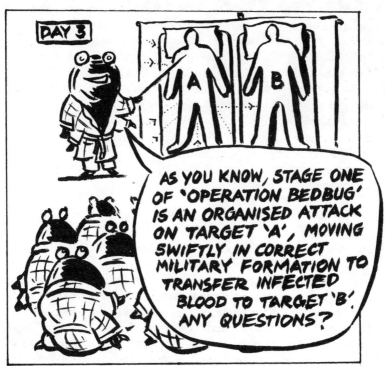

transmission while administering first aid. There have, however, been fears expressed by first-aiders of contracting HIV through mouth-to-mouth resuscitation, although there are no recorded cases of this occurring anywhere in the world and it is not regarded as a route of infection.

Any conceivable risk of HIV infection through mouth-to-mouth resuscitation would be due to contact with blood in the mouth, not saliva, which cannot transmit the virus. There are devices available to prevent mouth-to-mouth contact, but whether they are effective or necessary is still unclear. What is certain is that any possible risk of HIV infection through the presence of blood during mouth-to-mouth resuscitation is likely to be far smaller than the risk of causing harm by not providing emergency help to someone who needs it.

Dental Treatment

Dental equipment should always be sterilised to remove any possibility of HIV transmission through blood-to-blood contact. Dentists have strict guidelines to follow in preventing infection both to and from their patients: this covers the common cold virus and a range of other infections, not just HIV. Research on the possibility of HIV transmission to dentists through surgery on patients with the virus has repeatedly shown that dentists are not at risk if standard hygienic precautions are always followed. There is therefore no justification for dentists to refuse to treat people with HIV.

Swimming Pools and Jacuzzis

There are three reasons why swimming pools do not transmit HIV infection:

1. The water in the pool dilutes body fluids such as blood, making HIV transmission far more difficult.
2. Chlorine or other disinfectants in swimming pools inactivate the virus.
3. People do not often go swimming with open, bleeding cuts on their bodies (if they do, these should be covered with a dressing).

There are no cases of HIV transmission through sitting in a jacuzzi reported from anywhere in the world. Jacuzzis are safe in terms of HIV infection for the same reasons that swimming pools are, and the additional fact that water in a jacuzzi circulates rapidly provides another reason why this is not a route of HIV infection.

Sun Beds, Steam Rooms, and Saunas

Sweat has never been shown to transmit HIV effectively, as the virus is not present in the sweat of a person with HIV in enough quantities to cause infection. For this reason, sharing saunas, steam rooms or sun beds with a person with HIV is not a risk. If, however, saunas or steam rooms are also places where you have sex, Chapter 5 may be helpful.

Hairdressing, Ear-piercing and Cosmetic Treatments

Hot water and detergent both work to sterilise scissors and razors at the hairdressers quite adequately, and most establishments are likely to keep their equipment clean as a matter of course. In any case, the only conceivable risk of HIV at the hairdressers would be through having your skin pierced by a sharp object recently and thoroughly coated in the blood of a person with HIV. If you think your hairdresser is likely to behave in this manner, it may be time for a change.

Ear-piercing and some cosmetic treatments involve a theoretical HIV infection risk if blood is drawn and equipment shared without being properly sterilised. Many ear-piercing establishments now use a special instrument which injects a sterile stud and 'butterfly' clip into your ear. With this method it is the stud which pierces your ear, so there is no risk of contact with contaminated equipment. It should in any case be stressed that even where cosmetic equipment (for example, for ear-piercing or electrolysis) is re-used and inadequately sterilised, the amount of blood involved is likely to be tiny, so the risk is very limited.

There are no recorded cases of people being infected with HIV through undergoing cosmetic treatment of any kind. As stated above, increased training and information for workers in this field has led to much greater awareness of health and safety procedures. It is, however, always worth checking what measures are taken if you are concerned about this.

A Note about Blood

It is worth remembering that body fluids which do not transmit HIV, such as saliva, may become more infectious if they have traces

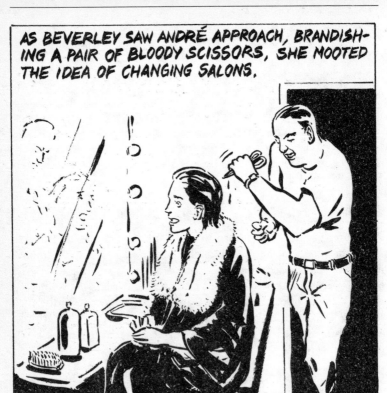

AS BEVERLEY SAW ANDRÉ APPROACH, BRANDISH-ING A PAIR OF BLOODY SCISSORS, SHE MOOTED THE IDEA OF CHANGING SALONS.

of infected blood in them. Although there are no recorded cases of HIV transmission through shared toothbrushes, it is probably sensible not to share if you, or the person with whom you are sharing, have bleeding gums or mouth ulcers. Similarly, sharing razors or scissors has never been shown to be a route of HIV transmission, but it would not be sensible to shave with a razor freshly coated in someone else's blood. In any case, blood-to-blood contact is risky not just in terms of HIV infection, but also for other viruses such as hepatitis B, which is far more easily transmitted than is HIV. Chapters 5 and 7 give more information about preventing HIV infection in domestic and other settings.

4

HIV NON-SEXUAL TRANSMISSION

The three most common routes by which HIV can be transmitted are unsafe penetrative sex; 'blood to blood' contact (situations which allow infected blood to get into your body); and from a mother with HIV to her child during or after pregnancy. Chapter 5 discusses safer sex; this chapter will look at avoiding risks from contact with infected blood, and the issues related to pregnancy.

Contact with infected blood may occur when a person is given a contaminated blood transfusion or blood products, through accidents where blood spillages occur, or when equipment to inject drugs is shared. More information on all these areas follows.

GIVING AND RECEIVING BLOOD

Since October 1985 all blood donated in Britain has been tested for antibodies to HIV, and in June 1990 testing also began for antibodies to the second type of the virus, HIV2 (see Chapter 2). People who have received blood since this screening programme began are well protected, because blood supplies are now very safe: if donated blood turns out to contain antibodies for HIV it will not be used. Furthermore, the National Blood Transfusion Service has asked people who think they have put themselves at risk from HIV infection not to donate blood. This additional precaution appears to have worked: the current risk of receiving infected blood in a transfusion has been estimated at about one in a million. It is also safe to donate blood, because all equipment used to take blood is sterile. There are therefore no grounds to refuse to donate or receive blood in Britain purely through fears of HIV infection.

If you give blood, your blood sample is tested for HIV antibodies. If the result is negative you will hear nothing more from the transfusion service, but if it is positive the sample will be tested again and you will be invited to attend the local centre. Your result should be given to you in confidence by a doctor, and counselling should be available; if not, you will be given details of organisations who can provide counselling and support. You will also be asked not to donate blood again.

It is not, however, a good idea to donate blood in order to find out whether or not you have HIV infection, because you will not be given any counselling or information before the test is taken, and so will not be prepared for the shock and distress a positive result can cause. You will also not be ready for other possible effects a test result, whether positive or negative, can have on your life. It is far better to arrange to have an HIV antibody test through a sexually transmitted disease clinic, because you will be offered counselling and information both before and after the test, if you decide to take it. Chapter 6 gives more information about the HIV antibody test and about what you need to think about before you decide whether or not to be tested.

This is the situation regarding giving and receiving blood in Britain. It does not necessarily apply elsewhere. If you are planning to travel or live abroad and are unsure of the precautions taken by other countries, it is worth getting information before you go. The Department of Health, the Medical Advisory Service for Travellers Abroad (MASTA) at the London School of Hygiene and Tropical Medicine or the appropriate embassy should give you more details. It is possible to buy medical packs containing sterilised injecting equipment and dressings to take with you. These are available from MASTA and elsewhere; see the Directory at the back of this book for further information.

Blood Products

Some people have become infected with HIV through receiving products made from contaminated blood. This is the case for a large number of people with haemophilia, an inherited disease which appears to affect men almost exclusively and which is the result of a shortage of proteins in the blood that help it to clot. Haemophilia A is the most common form of the disease and involves a lack of the blood protein Factor VIII. In the much rarer haemophilia B, Factor IX is what is missing. Symptoms of severe haemophilia include regular and acutely painful bleeding into muscles and joints, which can be fatal if left untreated.

Over the past 20 years it has become possible to produce Factors VIII and IX in storable forms, giving people with haemophilia the freedom to treat themselves at home on a regular basis and to have risk-free dental or medical surgery should they need it. The two main forms of both Factors VIII and IX available are a *cryoprecipitate* (prepared from small batches of blood donations) and a *concentrate* (mass-produced from large numbers of blood donations and involving a chemical process to separate out the factor needed). People with severe haemophilia who tend to need regular supplies of either factor are generally treated with concentrates. Both methods of production inactivate many potentially damaging agents in blood donations, but they do not inactivate viruses.

In the 1980s, most of the concentrated form of Factor VIII used in Britain was imported from the United States. HIV had been around in the US for some years, but because it was not discovered as the cause of AIDS until 1983, some of the blood donations used to prepare Factor VIII were infected with HIV. About half of the people with haemophilia who needed Factor VIII at that time became infected with the virus as a result. Factor IX, which has been produced mainly in Britain, caused far fewer infections because levels of HIV infection were far lower in the UK in the late 1970s and early 1980s than they were in the US. Factor VIII produced in this country also resulted in fewer infections, for the same reason.

Since HIV infection among people with haemophilia became apparent there have been two methods of preventing future infection risks. One is through decreasing use of concentrates, but this is mainly an option only for people with mild haemophilia or haemophilia B, who can use cryoprecipitates or plasma instead of concentrates. The second method is heat-treating, which is now an effective way of inactivating HIV in Factor VIII (Factor IX is less effectively heat treated).

Unfortunately, heat-treating of Factor VIII came too late for many people with haemophilia. Over 1,000 people were infected with HIV through contaminated imports in the late 1970s and early 1980s, and in 1988 a campaign was launched by the Haemophilia Society in London to get financial compensation from the British Government for those people. As already mentioned in Chapter 1, in late 1990, the Government announced a £42 million payment as compensation to people with haemophilia who had become infected with HIV through contaminated blood products. Previous payments amounting to £34 million were regarded as 'one off' amounts rather than compensation, and led to the setting up of a body called the MacFarlane Trust to administer monies to individuals on a special-needs basis.

Health and Safety Procedures

The following guidelines will be helpful for dealing with HIV infection risks in any setting, but may have particular relevance for those involved in health care. There is further information about practical health and safety measures in the home and elsewhere in Chapter 7.

In many cases, safety procedures discussed below may not appear to be anything special. That is because they do not need to be: generally, common-sense hygienic procedures are fully adequate to deal with HIV infection risks through spilled body fluids. It is worth remembering that even if it is not possible to stick to safety precautions exactly, the chances of HIV transmission are still pretty remote. The number of people known to have been infected with HIV in occupational settings is tiny, and has generally been the result of regular close contact with infected blood. The risk of HIV transmission even when exposure to infected blood has occurred is thought to be considerably less than 1 per cent. However, as in so many other areas, HIV and AIDS have tended to draw attention to shortcomings and inadequacies in general health and safety policy.

There is no evidence that spilled body fluids such as urine, vomit or faeces have ever transmitted HIV, and they are not generally considered to be routes of infection for the virus. Infected blood is likely to be far more dangerous as far as HIV transmission is concerned. However, these fluids should be treated with the same caution as blood, for two reasons. They may contain infected blood which could increase the risk of HIV transmission, and they may transmit other viruses and parasitic infections which could be harmful, particularly to a person whose immune system is already weakened by HIV infection.

Dealing with Spilled Body Fluids
- All spillages on surfaces should be dealt with promptly using a solution of one part bleach to ten parts water (as hot as possible). You can buy pre-diluted bleach, known as *Sodium Hypochlorite 1 per cent*, from the chemist; it can be used as it is, without water.
- Wear disposable latex gloves; if they are not available make sure you have covered open wounds with sticking plaster or bandage. This will protect your hands from the bleach as well as from the spillage. It is also a good idea to use disposable towels to clean up; if none are available leave the used cloth to soak in a similar

bleach solution. The hot wash of a washing machine is adequate to deal with spillages on clothing or bed linen.

- Any disposable items such as gloves, cloths or paper towels should be placed in a sealed bag and thrown away.

Needlestick Injuries

Accidents with needles and other sharp instruments (called 'needlestick' or 'sharps' injuries) are common in health care settings. Despite their frequency, by July 1990 there were only 19 cases identified world-wide of people infected with HIV through needlestick injuries in the workplace, out of a total of 37 cases world-wide of transmission through blood contact in workplace settings. This figure is not likely to be completely accurate, as up-to-date data depend on good reporting practices. It does however indicate that HIV transmission risks through workplace accidents are extremely low generally; the risk of infection through contact with a contaminated needle has been calculated at less than 0.5 per cent, or 1 in 200. Around 40 per cent of needlestick injuries occur when re-sheathing needles, so this should be avoided unless absolutely necessary.

- If you do accidentally jab yourself with a needle that someone else has used, clean the wound by squeezing it (but avoid sucking) to get blood flowing out, in the same way as you would with a cut that has become contaminated by dirt or another person's blood. Wash the wound carefully with soap and water, apply antiseptic and cover with a plaster.
- All sharps should be disposed of in a disposal box or bin which should be puncture-proof. Plastic ones are better than cardboard. If you are using needles regularly, keep the disposal bin near you and have it incinerated when it is full – this can be done in the hospital. Sharps bins should be disposed of when they are about three-quarters full.

Sterilising Equipment

Non-disposable items used, for example, during dental or medical surgery can be sterilised through heat-based methods or chemical disinfection (i.e. bleach or glutaraldehyde solution). HIV can be inactivated if the contaminated instrument is placed in an autoclave at a minimum of 115°C/239°F for 30 minutes, or at 160°C/320°F in a hot air oven for one hour.

Reducing Risk in the Workplace

Research indicates that, if not all, the vast majority of exposures to HIV in occupational settings are avoidable. (It should be noted that exposures through selling sex, which is also an occupation, are not included in this definition.) A study in San Francisco revealed that 60 per cent of workers took inadequate precautions to protect themselves, and research among American paediatricians showed that 70 per cent had jabbed themselves or been jabbed by needles with patients' blood on them.

Studies of workers in health care settings have pinpointed a lack of experience and information about safety procedures and infection control measures. In late May 1990, the British Medical Association issued a statement outlining a 'deplorable complacency' on the part of doctors and medical students in reporting needlestick injuries at work. John Dawson, head of the professional division of the BMA, stated that there could be as many as 1,000 accidental injuries with sharps occurring daily, and that the failure to report these could be due to inexperience as much as to work pressures.

This highlights the need for education and training programmes for carers and ancillary staff. Provision of detailed, written guidelines on infection control, means of dealing with waste disposal and handling sharps can go a long way to help prevent accidents in health centres, GP practices, laboratories, operating theatres, during home or maternity care and elsewhere. Staff who have to carry out the procedures should be involved in drawing up these guidelines and reviewing them; policies should not be bits of paper which just sit about forgotten on shelves or in filing cabinets. Monitoring of accidents is essential, because it may help to show how they can be avoided, and improved procedures can follow.

Infection control measures do not come cheap. Funding is required for training and education programmes as well as for supplies of protective equipment. The price of such measures is, however, arguably low in comparison with the enormous personal costs of HIV in terms of preventable transmission, discriminatory testing procedures and the distress and division these can generate.

A Note About Confidentiality

Confidentiality is about developing relationships on a basis of trust, and respecting the privacy and autonomy of individuals. It is a vital aspect of maintaining good work practice with regard to HIV infection and AIDS, applying not just to health care settings, but to offices, factories, schools, colleges and so on.

Good infection control procedures are essential to the success of maintaining confidentiality. Appearances and guesswork cannot tell you who has HIV infection; anyone may have it and be unaware of it. If good safety practice is taught and followed universally, there is no need for any individual's HIV antibody status to be disclosed for reasons of protecting others.

DRUG USE AND HIV

Why Drug Use is Risky

In the following section, the specific risks of HIV infection related to sharing equipment to inject drugs are discussed, as well as more general risks associated with drug use.

Like sex, taking drugs has always carried a degree of risk, but the arrival of HIV has increased the risks involved in sharing needles to inject drugs. When a drug is injected, it is first heated in water until it dissolves, then drawn up through a needle into a syringe. The drug is injected into a user's vein, then he or she may draw blood back from the vein into the barrel of the syringe to flush out whatever is left of the drug. This mixture of drug and blood is then injected back into the vein, so that the user can get a second 'hit' from the drug and make sure none of it is wasted.

If the user has HIV and the injecting equipment is shared, a small quantity of infected blood remaining behind in the barrel of the syringe could be injected by another user into his or her body along with the drug. This is a particularly effective way for HIV to be transmitted. As explained in Chapter 3, sharing mixing equipment such as a spoon, bowl or bottle top may also be risky, because traces of a person's blood could get onto it and be injected with the drug by another person. However, there is no evidence that this is a common route of infection for injecting drug users.

HIV infection is, however, only part of the risk involved with sharing equipment to inject drugs. Other serious infections can be passed on in this way, such as septicaemia and hepatitis B. There are also particular risks for drug injectors using impure drugs. Street drugs (as opposed to those obtained through a doctor's prescription) may be mixed or 'cut' with other substances such as chalk, brick dust or cleaning powder, which may lead to blocked veins, abscesses and other skin problems. For a person with HIV, use of impure drugs could strain his or her immune system further and lessen his or her ability to fight off other infections. Also, smoking cigarettes, marijuana or other drugs can damage the lungs, which in people with immune deficiency are often the first site of serious infections (see Chapter 2). There is further information on living with HIV and drug use in Chapter 7.

There are other reasons why taking any drugs may carry a risk of HIV transmission. Safer sex and using drugs may not go well together. Drugs can affect a person's judgement and make him or her lose sight of the risks of unsafe sex, or feel disinclined to think about ways of having sex more safely. Someone involved in sex work to pay for drugs may find it difficult to resist offers of drugs or increased payment in exchange for unsafe sex.

Why Safer Drug Use May Be Difficult

In general, it is likely that a person's ability to avoid HIV infection through injecting drugs is affected by a range of factors other than simply having the desire to do so and the right information. The amount of time and energy available to think about staying safe is important, in addition to the degree of support offered by friends or family, the level of dependency upon the drug, access to clean injecting equipment, and the availability of appropriate services. Poverty might also be an issue. It is cheaper to inject a drug than to sniff, smoke or swallow it. This is because the effect of an injected drug is much greater than the same quantity of that drug taken by any other method.

Concerns about having safer sex and not sharing equipment may seem pretty irrelevant to a drug user who is obliged to spend a great deal of time thinking about how to get money for the next supply of the drug. Similarly, a person who would not generally share works to inject may find that in a state of withdrawal, staying safe by not sharing someone's injecting equipment comes a long way behind meeting the immediate need for a hit.

Finally, people who share works with friends may worry that stopping sharing might be regarded as a sign of mistrust. It could imply that the person who does not want to share works thinks the other users have HIV. It could also imply that the person concerned has HIV. Even though wanting to stay safe or protect other people is not something to be ashamed of, such problems are often hard to sort out alone. If any of the difficulties discussed above apply to you, you may wish to get help. National organisations listed in the Directory at the back of this book can provide you with counselling, advice and information. They may also put you in touch with local drug services, if you want this.

Ways to Stay Safe

If you are sharing works to inject drugs, the following information may be useful to you. You may already be taking steps to stay safe from HIV infection, but if not, it might help to consider what changes you can realistically make.

- If you inject drugs, you could consider alternatives such as smoking, sniffing or swallowing them. Since there is no risk of infected blood from another person getting into your body this way, there is no risk of HIV infection. Some drug treatment agencies provide methadone as an oral substitute for heroin, for example.
- If you feel you are not able to stop injecting, it is absolutely vital to use new equipment. There are now syringe and needle exchange schemes which will give you new injecting equipment. Many also provide condoms and guidance on safer sex, if you want it. If there is no exchange scheme in your area, some chemists sell injecting equipment. Keeping a supply of new equipment means that you do not have to share works with anyone else.
- If for any reason you are unable to keep a supply of new equipment, the best thing is to make sure the works you do have are kept clean. They should be cleaned every time they are used: allowing yourself to be passed used works or passing on your own used equipment to anyone else is extremely risky.

    There are several different ways to keep injecting equipment clean. Don't forget that you need to clean mixing equipment as well: avoid sharing spoons, water, or anything else that has been used to mix drugs. It is possible to get vials of sterilised water for mixing purposes; they are available from syringe exchange schemes. You can also get them from most chemists, but you will need a prescription.

    You can use bleach to clean your works. Flush out the needle and the barrel of the syringe with undiluted household bleach, then rinse them thoroughly with cold water two to three times, and repeat the process. Be very careful that you do rinse the works properly; injecting yourself with bleach accidentally could be dangerous. Do not flush used bleach or water back into their original containers, and remember that bleach can lose its strength if it is kept too long, or left out in the sunlight. If you are unhappy about using bleach, you could try using washing-up liquid mixed with water instead, following the same procedure. However, while bleach inactivates HIV, washing up liquid only helps draw the blood out of the needle and syringe.

Another method is to flush the works through with cold water, take the syringe apart, place all the parts in boiling water and leave them to boil for five minutes. This method is not to be recommended, however, because of the likelihood of damage to the plastic parts of the equipment.

Cleaning your injecting and mixing equipment will help to reduce the risk of HIV infection through drug injection, but the only way to eliminate the risk altogether is to stop sharing equipment.

• Make sure you dispose of used works in a safe way. Do not leave injecting or mixing equipment around where other people could use it or have an accident with it. If you can, take your works to a syringe exchange. If this is not possible, put them in a tin with a properly fitting lid before throwing them away.

• If you are having sex, make sure it is safer sex (see Chapter 5 for more information). Even if you have not practised safer sex or safer drug use before, it is never too late to start.

Getting Help

Services available for drug users vary enormously throughout Britain, so it is important to decide what kind of support you may be looking for and where it is available (see the organisations listed in the Directory at the back of this book for more information). You may want to stop injecting or to get clean works so you can make injecting safer. You may also be interested in more information about HIV and AIDS, condoms for safer sex, HIV antibody testing, counselling and support, as well as general help and advice about drug use. The key sources of help on drug-use issues (including HIV-related matters) are discussed below. Unfortunately, services specifically for drug users with HIV-related illness are still extremely limited.

Services Providing Advice, Counselling and Information on Drug Use
These services can help you to talk through any aspects of drug use that may be worrying you. They can also refer you to other agencies which can help you to deal with drug-related problems.

If there are no drug advice, counselling and information services where you live, you can call a national organisation working in drug use or HIV issues (see the Directory at the back of this book for information) and ask for details of organisations that could help you with specific needs. These might be connected with finding appropriate housing, getting legal help and so on.

Advice, counselling and information services may be run by health authorities or by voluntary organisations. Although what they can offer will vary from one region to another, all should give a confidential service with some degree of practical support. This might, for example, include a needle and syringe exchange scheme (see *Needle and Syringe Exchanges*, below). Such services are very often the best place to contact initially because they can help you to decide what help you need and how to get it. They are sometimes called 'street agencies', because they aim to be friendly and easy to approach. They should be able to give information to the families and friends of drug users as well.

National Health Service
Your GP is generally the first person from whom to seek help within the NHS. However, while some GPs are non-judgemental and experienced in drug use issues, this is not true for all. If you find that your GP is insensitive or unwilling to help you, you may need to find yourself a new GP. Chapter 6 gives you more information on this.

If you are pregnant, or have a general health problem, it is important to let your GP know that you take drugs, as this could affect the treatment that you are given. Although many GPs may feel that, unless you want to stop taking drugs, there is little they can do to help other than provide general medical care and give advice, there may be a drug dependency unit (also called a centre or clinic) at a local hospital that can help.

Drug dependency units (DDUs) may need a letter of referral from an appropriate professional worker. This could be your doctor, or, say, a social worker or probation officer. You will probably have to wait a few weeks before you can get an appointment. Many DDUs, however, will now accept self-referrals.

Services offered by DDUs vary. Some may aim to help people stop using drugs temporarily, to reduce the amount they are taking, or to stop taking drugs altogether. For example, methadone, an oral substitute for heroin, may be prescribed over a period of time to enable a gradual process of withdrawal from drug use. Staff at DDUs are usually very experienced in dealing with drug problems, and most are able to provide help and support for drug users with HIV. They may treat users on an 'in-patient' or 'out-patient' basis, depending on the needs of the individual concerned.

Some health authorities have a community drug team. These may be linked to the DDU, or may be independent. They can offer advice, information and practical help: some will liaise with GPs, or provide home visits, for example.

Residential Rehabilitation Centres
These are places where drug users stay for periods ranging from a few months to several years. Residents are generally required to have stopped using drugs for at least 24 hours before they are admitted. While the approach, rules and accessibility of each type of scheme vary, all try to provide residents with the skills and confidence to lead a fulfilling life without drugs. Examples of such schemes tend to fall into four broad groups: community-based hostels, Christian-based hostels, therapeutic communities, and 'Minnesota method' schemes, which follow a 12-step programme towards abstinence.

There are a number of reasons why residential rehabilitation may not be appropriate for a drug user who is HIV symptomatic. Sometimes painkilling drugs may be essential for a person with HIV-related illness, and staff and other residents may find this problematic. Rehabilitation centres may also not be able to provide the medical care necessary for a person who is ill, and so the programme of abstinence they offer might be interrupted by periods in hospital. Some centres also require residents to carry out domestic tasks or attend regular meetings, which might be too tiring for a person who has HIV disease. It is important to find out as much as you can about any rehabilitation centre you are considering before making a commitment to it, particularly if you are a drug user with HIV illness. Drugs advisory services (see the Directory at the back of this book) can give you further information.

Currently, the ROMA project in London and Kaleidoscope in Richmond-upon-Thames are the only residential centres in the UK which take people who are still using drugs. City Roads in London is a centre for people in a drug-related crisis of any kind; it is the only one of its kind in the UK. Residents stay for a maximum of

21 days and are placed on a detoxification programme. At the end of that period they may either move on to another centre or return to the community.

Needle and Syringe Exchanges
These are places where you can dispose of used works safely and pick up clean equipment in exchange. They should operate on a completely confidential basis, and may be run by DDUs, community drug teams or voluntary organisations. Help, advice and counselling about HIV and AIDS may also be available, as well as free condoms and information about safer sex. Some chemists also run an exchange, or sell injecting equipment.

Self-help Groups
Unlike many gay men, drug users do not often have an identifiable community to whom they can turn for support and help. Self-help groups can provide this, and in some areas may be the only service available to drug users. They aim to offer emotional support and practical help both to users and to their families and friends. They can also provide a 'safe place' to air feelings, which may not be available elsewhere. Styles and approaches of self-help groups vary; you can get details of what is available in your area through drug advisory and information services, such as those listed in the Directory.

PREGNANCY AND HIV

Over the past five years, the HIV epidemic has had a serious impact upon women's health. Women of all ages make up an increasingly large proportion of people with HIV and AIDS globally: in major cities of regions as diverse as western Europe, the United States and sub-Saharan Africa, AIDS is now the primary cause of death in women aged 20 to 40 years. The World Health Organization predicted in July 1990 that around 3 million women world-wide with AIDS would die in the 1990s; about the same number of women of childbearing age are already thought to have HIV infection. Like men, women are at risk through sexual activity, through contact with infected blood and blood products, and through sharing equipment to inject drugs. Unlike men, many women have to deal with the dilemmas raised by pregnancy and childbirth.

Women with HIV may pass the virus to their baby before birth, or afterwards through breastfeeding (although there are still few cases of this). It is also possible, but quite unproven, that HIV may be passed from mother to baby *during* birth. For these reasons, an HIV-positive woman may be unwilling to run the risk of pregnancy. Another risk is the possibility of exposing her partner to infection if she has unsafe sex in order to get pregnant. An HIV-negative woman might risk HIV infection herself if her partner is HIV positive.

Whether you are HIV negative or positive, or unsure of your HIV antibody status, if you are planning to get pregnant in the future you may find the information in the following section of this book useful.

HIV Transmission from Mother to Child

Research into HIV transmission from mothers to babies is still inadequate, and many questions remain unanswered. However, studies conducted in Europe and elsewhere have shown that there are three possible routes by which HIV can be transmitted from mothers to children through pregnancy and childbirth.

1. The foetus may become infected in the womb, since HIV is able to cross the placenta during pregnancy.

    This is thought to be the most common way in which the virus is passed from HIV-positive mothers to babies. It is still unclear at what stage of pregnancy this may occur, although studies conducted in 1985 and 1986 revealed that the foetus may be infected at as early as 15 weeks into the pregnancy.
2. HIV transmission may also take place at birth, through the baby's contact with infected vaginal fluid and blood from the mother, although there is still no hard evidence that this occurs, and far less is known about it than about transmission during pregnancy. If conclusive evidence of HIV transmission at birth were provided, issues about the best mode of delivery could be given fuller attention, and the chances of preventing HIV transmission from mother to baby would substantially increase. As it is, there is not enough information to show that one mode of delivery is better than another in preventing HIV transmission at birth.
3. Finally, the mother may pass HIV to her baby during breastfeeding, through infected breastmilk. This route of transmission is, however, quite rare, though a recent study established that it can take place. Mothers with HIV in Britain are

advised to bottlefeed rather than breastfeed their babies. However, in countries where it may be harder to get alternative sterilised supplies of milk and where infant deaths from chronic diarrhoea may be higher than from HIV, women are still advised to breastfeed their babies whether or not they have HIV infection. Breastmilk supplied in British hospitals is safe because it is pasteurised (thereby inactivating HIV); HIV-positive women are asked not to donate breastmilk.

Detecting HIV Infection in Babies

It is impossible to tell at birth whether or not a mother with HIV has passed the virus to her baby. This is because a baby automatically inherits from his or her mother the antibodies she has in her bloodstream (antibodies develop in the body as a response to a vast range of infections, including HIV). If the mother has HIV infection, the baby will inherit her antibodies to HIV even though he or she may not actually be infected by the virus. As stated in Chapter 2, the HIV antibody test does not detect the presence of HIV itself in the bloodstream; it detects the presence of *antibodies* to HIV. This means that a baby whose mother has HIV will always produce a positive HIV antibody test result, whether or not he or she actually has HIV infection, because the test will detect the mother's antibodies to HIV that are still in the baby's bloodstream.

For this reason, it is not possible to be sure about a baby's HIV antibody status until he or she is around 18 months of age, because that is how long it generally takes before the baby's blood has lost the maternal antibodies. (In exceptional cases, some babies may develop their own antibodies at 12 months, while others may not do so until 22 months.) Babies with HIV infection have generally developed their own antibodies to the virus by this time, so a test result is far more likely to be accurate. Even so, clinics caring for babies and young children of mothers with HIV usually prefer to test repeatedly for infection: sometimes antibodies to infection may take longer to develop, and in a very few cases may disappear altogether in a baby with HIV. There is still not enough research into this area to clarify why this may occur. Generally, babies of mothers with HIV are monitored very carefully for signs of HIV-related illness and a weakened immune system; Chapter 2 gives more information about medical treatments, and Chapter 8 more about caring for a child with HIV infection or AIDS.

When it first became clear that pregnant women with HIV could pass the virus to their babies, it was also assumed that getting pregnant could cause HIV-positive women to develop severe immune deficiency and HIV-related illness more quickly. This is because pregnancy tends to weaken the immune system in order that the mother's body will not reject the foetus. This view is not supported by medical evidence, however; there is therefore little reason to be afraid that getting pregnant will make you become ill more quickly if you have HIV infection.

There are other questions related to HIV infection and pregnancy which still require answers. It remains unclear, for example, whether having HIV infection is likely to mean your pregnancy will be more difficult or painful. However, research suggests that there is little difference in health during pregnancy between women who are HIV negative and women with HIV but no signs of related illness ('HIV asymptomatic').

There is no evidence as yet that the number of pregnancies a woman with HIV has increases the risk of passing the virus to her baby. It *is* clear, however that an HIV-positive mother may give birth to a baby with HIV infection and later give birth to a child who is HIV negative; it may also work the other way round. What is also, unfortunately, evident is that babies with HIV have a fairly strong chance of becoming ill and developing AIDS more rapidly than do adults with HIV. This is because in a baby or young child the immune system is less developed than that of an adult; infections such as HIV therefore pose a far greater risk. Findings from a European study of children born to women with HIV suggest that one in three HIV-positive children will develop AIDS in their first six months and nine out of ten will develop symptoms of illness after two years.

The prognosis for a child with HIV, as for an adult, depends to a great extent on economic and environmental factors. In countries where resources for health care and drug treatments are limited, children with HIV may become seriously ill or die without receiving medical attention. Poverty plays a significant role in this. Unsanitary living conditions, poor nutrition and exposure to other prevalent infections can severely shorten the life of both children and adults with HIV infection.

If you have HIV and you have a baby or young child who does not have the virus, remember that ordinary care, love or affection will not put him or her at risk. Hugging, kissing, tickling and cuddling your baby are all safe. In the same way, if your child does have HIV then he or she does not pose a risk to other members of your family nor to friends. There is no reason for a baby or child with HIV to be kept away from other children. He or she should be allowed to lead as ordinary a life as health will allow.

Assessing the Risks

There is no way of knowing for certain whether or not you will pass HIV to your baby if you are pregnant and have the virus. If you are in a heterosexual relationship and you plan to get pregnant, you might infect your partner through unsafe sex if you have HIV and he does not, or, if he is HIV positive, he might pass the virus to you. Donor insemination techniques may be helpful for couples wishing to have a baby where one partner is HIV positive; they can similarly be useful for lesbian couples who want to have a baby (see *Insemination by Donor*, below).

Above all, it is important to know that the chance of an HIV-positive pregnant woman infecting her baby is much smaller than was originally thought. As stated in Chapter 3, when studies were first conducted into rates of HIV transmission between HIV-positive women and their babies, it appeared that there was a 50 per cent likelihood of passing the virus on. Current studies in Europe, however, suggest that the risk of transmission is considerably lower, at around 20 per cent.

There are several reasons for this difference. The earliest studies involved women who were already ill with HIV-related diseases; they were considered to be much more likely to infect their babies because levels of HIV appear to be higher in the blood of people who are at a late stage of infection and developing symptoms of illness than in people who are HIV asymptomatic. Research suggests therefore that HIV asymptomatic women are less likely to pass HIV infection to their babies. Levels of HIV infection in the blood are similarly thought to be high around the time of infection; this means that pregnant women who have just become infected may have a greater risk of passing the virus to their babies than pregnant women who have had HIV infection for some time, but no symptoms of illness.

If you have HIV infection and want to have a baby, the best thing to do is get all the information and advice you can, and to remember that the decision about whether or not to get pregnant, or (if you are already pregnant) whether or not to have the baby must lie with you. No one else can make up your mind for you, and it is important that you do not allow yourself to be persuaded or pushed into making a decision with which you are unhappy. There are organisations listed in the Directory at the back of this book which can provide you with further help and advice; counselling and support are also available if you want them.

In making your decision you may need to consider your own state of health and the risk of the baby becoming infected, getting ill and possibly dying. You may need to think about possible feelings of trauma and guilt if your baby does have HIV infection, and how you might cope with these. It might be helpful to ask yourself questions about where and how to get support in coping with the challenges posed by looking after a baby with HIV. Friends, your sexual partner(s), and other women in a similar situation may be able to help and support you. If you decide to have a baby, you will need proper medical care and attention to make sure that you stay healthy and that the pregnancy progresses properly.

Insemination by Donor

Getting pregnant through donor insemination is an option for women who do not have HIV and who are unsure of their partner's antibody status, or who know that their partner has HIV infection. It is also an option in couples where a man is HIV negative and a woman HIV positive, because the male partner may be able to donate his sperm to the woman without risking infection from her.

Lesbians and single women may also want to use donor insemination services; however, some clinics in Britain offer services only to married women. In that situation, you may need to make your own arrangements with a donor whom you know to be HIV negative (and he will need to take an HIV antibody test to be certain of this, or to have taken a test recently and practised safer behaviour ever since). Further advice about organising donor insemination without using a clinic is available from some of the organisations listed in the Directory at the back of this book.

All donors at clinics (whether National Health Service or private) have to take an HIV antibody test before they can give sperm. Make sure that the clinic you use double-checks the initial test result. This can be done by storing and freezing the donated sperm until the donor has taken a second test a few months after the first (it generally takes around three months after the date of infection for antibodies to HIV to develop). The man donating the sperm is meant to stay safe from HIV infection risks during this period, and you must be careful to do so as well.

There has been limited research into treating semen from men with HIV so that the seminal fluid (which in an HIV-positive man generally contains the virus) can be separated from the sperm (which does not generally contain the virus). This would enable the female partner of a man with HIV to become pregnant through donor insemination techniques using her partner's semen, without becoming infected with HIV at the same time. However, there is still no evidence that any procedure can reliably remove HIV from semen.

Pregnant Women and HIV Antibody Testing

Pregnant women face risks other than HIV infection. They may also be at risk of being pushed into accepting an HIV antibody test that they do not need or want. Pregnancy is a highly emotive state, and pregnant women may be more than usually vulnerable to pressure, particularly where the health of their future baby is concerned. However, coercion has never been a sound guiding principle for good health care. Medical practitioners who do not allow women to choose whether or not to be tested for HIV antibodies, or to proceed with pregnancy if they have HIV infection, are ignoring some important facts.

Women who may feel stigmatised by drug use, poverty or lack of educational qualifications might see motherhood as the one time when they have a sense of self-worth. In some societies, a woman's social status is dependent on motherhood. The risks of HIV infection to mother and child through pregnancy might not change this. Denying women choice in matters of pregnancy and health care could be disastrous: if women are uncomfortable with the services on offer, they will avoid them. In the long term, this could mean far more unwanted babies with HIV, and far more HIV-positive women receiving no medical attention or support. It could also mean that women who are HIV negative do not get the information and advice they need to stay safe from infection.

Some antenatal clinics actively encourage pregnant women to have an HIV antibody test. If you are in this situation, there are several things to bear in mind. No one has any legal right to force you to have an HIV antibody test if you do not want to do so. You could ask for information about what the test may mean for you (Chapter 6 of this book may be of help to you here). It also helps to make sure that, if you do decide to have the test, you will be offered counselling both before and afterwards. You may want to change your mind. On the other hand, if after counselling you still want to have the test, you need to be prepared for the fact that you could turn out to be HIV positive. Whether you agree to take the test or not should make absolutely no difference to the degree of support and help that the clinic offers you.

In January 1990 a nation-wide 'anonymous' testing programme (also called anonymous screening) was launched. This programme allows clinics to test for HIV antibodies in blood samples which have been taken for other purposes. The point of the anonymous testing programme is to get a clearer idea of how many people in Britain have HIV. One research study which resulted from this programme found that 1 in 500 pregnant women in London was HIV positive. Some health care professionals consider that relying entirely on figures based on 'voluntary testing' (i.e. people who decide to take the HIV antibody test for personal reasons) does not provide an up-to-date picture of how widespread the virus is. Chapter 6 gives more information about why this is, and about how anonymous testing works.

A variety of clinics now undertake anonymous testing. If you are visiting a clinic, it should be made clear to you if this is the clinic's policy. If there is an anonymous testing programme underway, it does not mean that *every* blood sample taken will be tested for HIV. It means that if your blood is taken for other tests, it *may* also be tested for HIV infection. You will not be given the result of the test, because the blood cannot be traced back to you. However, remember that you have the right to tell the clinic that you do not want your blood to be tested in this way. If you say nothing, it will probably be assumed that you are happy with the arrangement.

There is a great deal that remains unknown about mother-to-baby transmission of HIV. It is the least understood mode of HIV transmission, a point which is all the more alarming when we consider that the World Health Organization expects between 25 to 30 million women and children to be infected with HIV by the year 2000.

The many unanswered questions may relate to the fact that in the early years of the HIV epidemic in the West, far more men were affected by the virus than were women (although in some developing countries, men and women have been equally affected by HIV since the epidemic began). It may also be due to the status of many of the women already infected. Women who use drugs, Black and Hispanic women, women who are involved in prostitution or whose poverty may, in some countries, make health care inaccessible to them tend not to be seen as priorities by governments funding research and health services. In many ways, lack of information about HIV and pregnancy is another example of how women's health needs in general have been ignored or neglected world-wide.

5

LOVING CAREFULLY

Still, love is possible.
– *Pushkin*

SAFER SEX AND YOU

Trainers running workshops on HIV and AIDS sometimes ask participants to play a word game exploring their attitudes to sex in general and safer sex in particular by writing down words they associate with each. One of the key differences between the two lists produced by this exercise is that words linked with sex are often much more positive and varied than those linked with safer sex. Where terms such as 'pleasure', 'fun', 'sharing', 'intimacy', 'orgasm' and 'love' may crop up on the list for sex in general, they tend to feature far less frequently on the safer sex list. According to this exercise, staying safe from HIV leads many people to think of sex in a rather mechanical, restrictive context: words like 'spermicide', 'condom', 'lubricant', 'restriction', 'caution' and 'abstinence' are regularly mentioned.

It's clear from this that for many people there is a vast difference between their feelings about sex and about safer sex. Yet the difference between what is safe and what is unsafe is nothing like as great as one might think. The only sexual activity that has been proved to be definitely unsafe in terms of HIV infection is penetrative sex (penetration of the penis into the vagina or anus) without a condom, which is considered to be the most common cause of HIV infection world-wide.

How important the difference between sex and safer sex is for you depends on what you think of as sex. For some people, penetrative sex may appear to be the only way to have 'real' sex: if that is so, all other types of sexual activity can be relegated to the realm of 'foreplay', and ideas about safer sex may focus entirely on using condoms during penetration. This is significant not just because it may limit the enjoyment and satisfaction that sex gives us, but also because research suggests that a majority of women may not reach orgasm through penetration alone. However, people who enjoy a range of sensual and sexual activities, such as stroking, kissing, masturbation and oral sex as well as penetration, may well find safer sex to be more liberating than restrictive.

Our view of sex is determined by what we know, what we enjoy, what we feel comfortable with and how important we want it to be. Our thoughts and feelings about it are shaped by our school education, what we have learned from our family and friends, cultural and religious beliefs, the political climate (civil rights legislation in particular), media messages and previous sexual experience.

Expectations play an important role, too. Your view of how important it is for you or for your partner to have one or several orgasms, to communicate your feelings and needs, to be seen as sexually experienced and capable, or conversely to take a passive role in case you appear too keen or 'knowledgeable' - these are all going to be important factors in what you make of safer sex.

The view that safer sex is simply doing less with fewer people is a myth sustained in part by British media messages about safer sex, which have tended to focus almost exclusively on either saying 'no' to sex altogether or on using condoms. It also relates to the view that there are certain prescribed patterns of sexual behaviour for heterosexuals, bisexuals, gay men and lesbians. For example: heterosexuals never indulge in anal sex, gay men do nothing else, and lesbians don't have much sex at all because lesbianism is a last resort for women who can't get a man.

Such ideas are obvious nonsense. They are dangerous not just because they are inaccurate and insulting, but because the general assumption that sexual identity automatically confers a hard and fast code of sexual behaviour only serves to confine us. There are no neatly labelled pigeonholes, no closed compartments. There is only a wide range of erotic possibilities, some of which you may enjoy and feel comfortable with and some of which may turn you off entirely. A person who is lucky enough to live in a society which allows it can choose the kinds of sex he or she has, and with whom. We don't have to like the sexual preferences of others, but we can decide to treat them with the respect we would like accorded to our own.

Finally, you might feel that safer sex is planned sex and therefore somehow unromantic, unexciting, unloving even. There is a vast array of literature to support this theory. In Mills and Boon romances, the appearance of the word 'condom' is as unlikely as is the chance that you or I are to be made Prime Minister. During the habitual surging tide of passion which sweeps all deserving heroines into the urgent embrace of prototypes such as Clint (fresh-faced but fully-formed boy next door) or Father Patrick (lapsed Catholic priest), going with the moment is all. There is little opportunity to break off for a second and fish about in your handbag or jacket pocket for a pack of *Durex Fetherlite*.

Spontaneity is synonymous with passion, planning ahead its opposite – or so we are led to believe. Perhaps that's a factor in the embarrassment some people may experience in discussing sex with partners, buying and carrying condoms – being seen to be prepared for the possibility of sex. Of course we plan and prepare for sex all the time, whether or not this is acknowledged. Sex doesn't 'just happen', we *make* it happen (unless we are pressured or coerced). Safer sex is no different. Anybody who wants to stay safe or, if HIV positive, to protect partners from infection, needs to think ahead, to communicate his or her feelings and to be as well-informed as possible about the options available.

Choosing safer sex need not prevent your relationships from being pleasurable, rewarding and exciting. In fact, quite the opposite. Safer sex offers the possibility for exploring and getting pleasure from our entire bodies, not just those parts that are generally labelled 'erogenous zones'. It can involve a greater degree of sensuality and intimacy with partners than we might have considered possible, using the full range of erotic experience offered to us by our five senses. By removing the possible tension and stress associated with sexual risk-taking, it may turn out to be much more enjoyable sex than unsafe sex. It is certainly likely to be better for our health.

Sex has always been a risky business. Fears about expressing our sexuality, about pregnancy and sexually transmitted diseases saw to that long before HIV arrived. These risks may have put people off but they have not succeeded in stopping people from having sex and enjoying it. Neither should HIV. Safer sex is still one of the most immediate preventive measures we have against the virus; as stated in Chapter 2, an effective vaccine against the virus is a long-term solution only, unlikely to be available for some years.

WHAT IS SAFER SEX?

Safer sex is any kind of sexual activity that reduces the risk of HIV passing between sexual partners. That means that if you are having a safer sexual relationship and you are HIV positive, you are taking care not to pass HIV on. It is worth remembering also that even if both you and your partner are already HIV positive, there is still a reason to have safer sex. You may put yourself at risk of other sexually transmitted infections if you do not, some of which may cause serious illness in people with already weakened immune systems. Since there are a number of different strains of HIV, a person with HIV could also be vulnerable to infection by another form of the virus, possibly resulting in increased damage to the immune system (see Chapter 2). If you are HIV negative, safer sex can protect you from possible infection by your partners.

It is not always possible to state categorically whether a particular sexual activity is 100 per cent safe or not: that's why the term *safer* sex rather than *safe* sex is used here. Once you are familiar with the basic, limited ways in which HIV is able to pass from one person to another, you are in a position to weigh up the risks for yourself.

HIV may be transmitted sexually when infected blood, semen or vaginal fluids from one person get into the body of his or her partner. The key point about safer sex is that infected body fluids from your partner should not be able to get into your body (or from you to your partner's body) through the skin of the penis, through the inside of the vagina or anus, through ulcers or sores in your mouth, or through open, uncovered cuts and wounds.

Keep sexual fluids and blood away from each other's genitals. If you have other sexually transmitted diseases such as genital ulcers, you may be more vulnerable to HIV infection, because they can act as a point of entry for the virus into your bloodstream. Bruising or cuts on the penis or inside the vagina can also increase the risk, for the same reason. It is important for the sake of good health generally to make sure sexual infections are treated immediately, as most can be easily cleared up at an early stage. Regular cervical smears for women and check-ups for men can help achieve this, and are similarly important for the health of men and women who are HIV positive.

Using condoms during penetrative sex will substantially reduce the risk of transmitting not just HIV, but most other sexual infections (see *Safer Condom Use*, below).

There is strong evidence from studies of couples where one

partner has HIV that women may be more vulnerable than men to infection through unsafe penetrative sex (see Chapter 3). Far more research is needed in this area, but women are increasingly significant in HIV and AIDS statistics; in some African countries, for example, there are as many women as men with HIV infection. This is likely to have an important impact upon health, education and support services both now and in the long term, but it should not distract us from the fact that both men and women are at risk from unsafe sex. Complacency is a highly dangerous substitute for safer behaviour.

Although HIV has been found in laboratory research to be present in other body fluids of an infected person – such as rectal secretions, urine, faeces, and breastmilk – this does not mean that the virus can be transmitted by these fluids. It has never, for example, been found to be transmitted by saliva, probably because it is rarely found to be present in the saliva of an infected person and, where it is present, it is in such small quantities that HIV transmission cannot occur.

Similarly, there is no risk of HIV transmission through contact with urine or faeces, although it is possible to pick up other infections from them, such as hepatitis B. It is worth bearing this in mind, because even if the kind of sex you have does not involve deliberate contact with urine or faeces, it may be difficult to avoid accidental contact, even if you and your partner have washed thoroughly before and after sex. If you have HIV infection and a weakened immune system, the infections which can arise from urine and faeces could have a significant effect on your health. For these reasons, it is sensible to treat them with caution.

Don't forget that the skin on your body, and your partner's body, is an excellent barrier to HIV. That's why hugging, cuddling, stroking and activities which do not allow infected body fluids to get into another person's body all form part of safer sex. If you follow this basic rule, and make sure cuts or wounds on your body are covered with a sticking plaster or bandage, you will find that there is a large range of activities that can play a part in your safer sex life.

WHAT IS UNSAFE SEX?

Unsafe sex is sex which is based on guesswork and false assumptions. Despite popular press representations of people with HIV and AIDS as wheelchair-bound skeletons on the brink of death, it is impossible to tell from appearances alone who has and has not got HIV infection.

Running through a checklist with your partner about sexual and medical history is not likely to be adequate protection against HIV. Neither is sticking to having sex among a closed circle of friends and contacts. It may help in sexual negotiations to know, like and trust the people you have sex with, but unfortunately this will not protect you from HIV infection if you are taking risks. The current state of the HIV epidemic in Britain is such that most people with HIV do not know that they have the virus. That could include your lover; it could include you.

Cutting down on numbers of sexual partners may lessen the chances of having sex with a person with HIV, but it will not make sex entirely safe. Safer sex with ten different people is safer than unsafe sex with one, if you do not know whether or not you, or that person, has HIV.

Unsafe sex is, in any case, not just sex that puts you or others at risk of HIV infection. It is *any* sex that you do not want to have, into which you may feel pressurised or coerced. Learning about what you enjoy sexually, and acquiring the negotiation skills to develop this with your partner, may be of some use in keeping sex safer for you psychologically as well as physically.

PRACTISING SAFER SEX

Safer Sex on Your Own

Being celibate, or choosing not to have sex with other people offers protection against sexual HIV infection because you are not in contact with another person's infected semen, blood, or vaginal fluid. (However, as stated above, you are still not safe from HIV if you share works to inject drugs.) There are all sorts of reasons why you may choose celibacy, but it is very important that you do not make that choice simply through fear of HIV infection. There is no need to avoid sex completely because you are worried about the risk of sexually transmitted disease - that is what safer sex is all about.

Staying with the Same Partner

Monogamy means different things to different people. It may imply staying with one partner for life, or it may mean sticking to one partner for as long as the relationship lasts, then having another relationship and sticking with that one person until it ends, and so on. This is sometimes called *serial monogamy*.

However you interpret it, monogamy offers no watertight guarantee against HIV infection. If you or your partner are infected and are not having safer sex, monogamy will not prevent HIV transmission. A monogamous relationship where one or both partners shares drug injecting equipment with other people is similarly unsafe.

Monogamy is, in any case, not a realistic option for some people. Relationships begin and end for all kinds of reasons, and the chances are that the first person you have a sexual relationship with is not necessarily going to be someone with whom you want to spend the rest of your life. Also, some people do not see monogamy as an option simply because they do not want to be limited to sex with one person.

Safer Sex: Checking it Out

The activities below could all form part of safer sex, bearing in mind the basic guidelines given above in *What is Safer Sex?* Please note that this list is not comprehensive by any means; with further information and your imagination you can build on it to suit yourself and your partner.

- Masturbation on your own (this is safe because you cannot pass infected semen or vaginal secretions to anyone else)
- Masturbation with your partner
- Kissing, licking, rubbing and stroking each other's bodies ~ such as the inner thighs, armpits, backs, behind the knees, back of the neck and so on
- Deep kissing ('French' kissing) ~ safest if you don't have bleeding gums or open mouth ulcers
- Sucking nipples, fingers, toes, and earlobes
- Showering together
- Hugging, cuddling, massage (this can be particularly nice with scented massage oils)
- Patting and spanking (but not if you do it so hard that you draw blood)
- Vaginal penetration, if he has a condom on his penis ~ see *Safer Condom Use* below for more details
- Anal penetration, if he has a condom on his penis ~ see *Safer Condom Use*, below

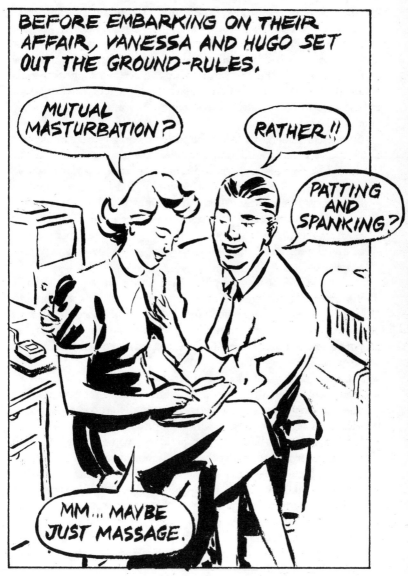

- Other types of penetration – The linings of your mouth, vagina and anus are far more sensitive than the intact skin on your body. This means that putting, for example, a finger with a cut on it into your partner carries a possible risk for you (because infected body fluids could get into your cut) or for your partner (because infected blood from your cut could get through the linings of your partner's mouth, vagina or anus). You can avoid these risks by covering open cuts with waterproof plaster, and by keeping your finger- and toenails short. It is not a good idea to put anything that has been in the anus directly into the vagina, as this can lead to bladder and vaginal infections such as cystitis and thrush.

If you are penetrated by someone else's fingers or toes, they should not have vaginal fluid or semen from that person on them (if it is *your* semen or vaginal fluid, don't worry ~ you cannot pass HIV to yourself). Similarly, whatever you put into your partner should not have your own body fluids on it. Putting your whole hand in the anus or vagina (fisting) is risky if it precedes or follows intercourse, because sensitive membranes may be torn, leading to bleeding. This makes it easier for a whole range of infections, not just HIV, to be transmitted to the person being penetrated. Some chemists sell disposable surgical gloves, which may give helpful protection.

These guidelines also apply to penetration by sex toys such as vibrators. Sharing these is dangerous, as infected secretions can be passed between you and your partner, and sex toys are often difficult to clean effectively. There is no danger if you and your partner have a vibrator each, for example, and do not swap these around.

- Sharing sexual fantasies. Your brain is the most powerful sex organ you have, and discussing situations that turn you on with your partner may be exciting for you, as well as completely safe. Two words of caution here, however: discussing fantasies may be safe, but acting them out is not if it involves risky sex. The information given here should guide you on this.

  Secondly, you need to feel sure that both you and your partner feel comfortable with and trust each other enough to share your sexual fantasies. Feelings of jealousy, embarrassment and shock are quite possible if the fantasies involve other people or activities you do not feel comfortable with. Remember that fantasy is just that; it does not mean that you necessarily want the situations or activities you imagine to actually happen to you, and the same goes for your partner.

- Oral sex ~ cunnilingus (kissing, licking and sucking a woman's clitoris and vulva). There is a possible risk of transmission if blood and large amounts of vaginal fluids get into the mouth. It is always the person whose mouth is involved (the active partner) who is at risk, which means that cunnilingus may be risky during menstruation (a woman's period), or if the active partner has bleeding gums or mouth ulcers. However, as large amounts of vaginal fluid do not usually get into the mouth during cunnilingus, it is generally not considered to be as risky as taking semen into the mouth. It may be safer to use a latex barrier if you are unhappy about the risk when you or your partner is menstruating (see *Safety with Latex - Barriers, or 'Dental Dams'*, below).

- Oral sex - fellatio (kissing, licking and sucking a man's penis). The risk of transmission comes from infected semen or pre-ejaculate (the fluid that comes out of the penis before a man ejaculates) getting into the active partner's mouth, particularly if he or she has bleeding gums or mouth ulcers. It is probably safer, therefore, if the man does not ejaculate ('come') in your mouth. Another possibility may be to use a condom in fellatio.

  There are so few recorded cases of HIV being transmitted through oral sex that it is certainly likely to be much safer than penetrative sex without a condom. However, as discussed above, the theoretical risks remain, and so it is sensible to try to make it as safe as possible.

- Licking and kissing your partner's anus (rimming) is not likely to transmit HIV, but may be a source of other infections if you get faeces in your mouth. Again, latex barriers may be helpful here (see *Safety with Latex - Barriers, or 'Dental Dams'*, below).

Safety with Latex - Condoms

A condom (rubber, johnnie or french letter) is a thin latex sheath which fits over the man's penis so that semen stays inside it and does not make contact with the mouth, vagina or anus during sex. Condoms have been used for years to prevent unwanted pregnancy, and are also an effective barrier against sexually transmitted diseases such as gonorrhoea, syphilis, cervical cancer, herpes and HIV infection.

Safer Condom Use
HIV, like semen, is not able to pass through intact rubber. However, condoms are only reliable in protecting against HIV infection if they do not break or slip off the penis during sex. If you know how to use them correctly, the chances of this are substantially reduced. It is also important to use them consistently: condoms are not going to offer you much protection against HIV if you only use them on an occasional basis.

Condoms with the British Standard Kitemark are tested for strength and reliability by manufacturers, but the standard allows one in every 125 condoms to fail the tests. This means that condoms cannot quite offer 100 per cent protection. Despite this, using a condom is certainly much safer than having anal or vaginal intercourse without one, and they are far more likely to fail as a result of incorrect use than from faulty production. Condoms are also good news for women, because unlike the contraceptive pill or coil they do not present any health risks.

Some people find the idea of using a condom off-putting because you have to stop to take it out of the packet and put it on, which may seem like an unwanted interruption to your lovemaking. But using condoms does not have to be a distraction from sexual activity; you can make it part of the fun and pleasure of sex, by using your imagination. Getting your partner to put the condom on for you, or seeing if you can put it on him without using your hands, are two ways to do this. If you keep a supply near to hand whenever and wherever you know you are likely to have sex, this will avoid a lengthy search at the last minute.

How to Put One On and Take it Off

Putting on and taking off a condom sounds simple, and it is. The guidelines below will help to avoid accidents with condom use.

- Make sure that the vagina or anus is well-lubricated. Water-based lubricant inside and around the vagina or anus will help prevent condoms from tearing or slipping off, and may also make sex more pleasurable for both of you (see *Lubricants and Spermicides,* below).
- Tear the condom packet open carefully, taking care that you don't damage the rubber with long fingernails or jewellery.
- Place the rolled-up condom on the end of the erect penis, making sure that you have got it the right way out so that it will roll down properly (the roll of rubber should be facing outwards).
- Roll the condom down the penis, squeezing the tip of the rubber between your thumb and finger to get rid of trapped air (some condoms have a teat to hold the semen). Putting a dab of water-based lubricant inside the tip of the condom beforehand helps to keep the air out, and may also improve sensation for the man (see *Lubricant and Spermicides,* below).
- If it feels as though the penis is getting soft during sex, either partner can try holding on to the base of the condom. This not

only helps keep the condom in place, it can be a nice feeling for the man whose penis it is.

- After sex, it may help to hold the condom on at the base of the penis when it is withdrawn from the vagina or anus. This stops the condom from coming off inside the other person and prevents spillage of semen. Either partner can roll the condom off the penis carefully, tie a knot in it and throw it away.

- Always use a new condom every time you have vaginal or anal intercourse, and keep your supply of condoms away from strong heat and sunlight, which may weaken the rubber.

- If you find putting a condom on yourself or your partner awkward and fiddly the first times you try, don't forget that practice makes perfect. Men can practise putting a condom on and taking it off when they masturbate, and you could also practise rolling a condom on and off a vibrator, for example (some people prefer to practise with carrots or other suitably-sized vegetables!) Improving your technique when you're on your own and not flustered by the feeling of needing to get it on as quickly and smoothly as possible could be enormously helpful in reducing any embarrassment and awkwardness you may feel about using condoms.

Condom Choice

You can find condoms in an enormous range of colours, designs, sizes, smells and even flavours. They range from the simple – your standard, pale pink, smooth-surfaced model – to the outrageous – knobbly-textured, multicoloured, peppermint-flavoured – whatever you want.

Condoms are available from supermarkets, shops, slot machines in toilets, garages, in chemists, and by mail order. You can also get them free from family planning clinics (whether you are male or female), and there is currently a campaign underway to enable patients to get them on prescription from their GP.

When choosing condoms you need to think about factors such as the way they smell or taste. This matters particularly if you use them during oral sex, although you can make them taste more pleasant by smearing them with flavoured yoghourts, for example. (Be careful of oil or acid in food or drink, which may damage the rubber.) You also need to consider factors such as how easy a particular condom is to put on, how it feels during sex, how much it costs, and so on. It's largely a question of experimenting until you and your partner find a brand that you enjoy and are happy with.

Look for the British Standard Kitemark on condom packets. Other condoms may have passed strict tests in the country of manufacture but are not kitemarked as they are imported. The kitemark only guarantees the condoms for vaginal sex, not anal sex, although some manufacturers now make thicker condoms that may offer more protection in anal sex. As the anus tends to be tighter and drier than the vagina, you will need to use a water-based lubricant to reduce friction on the condom (see *Lubricant and Spermicides*, below).

When you buy condoms, always check the sell-by date on the packet. If the condoms are too old for use they are more likely to tear or break during sex.

Safety with Latex – Barriers, or 'Dental Dams'

Latex barriers are sheets of thin rubber about five inches square, and, as they were originally developed for use in dental surgery, are also called 'dental dams'. Like condoms, they come in a range of

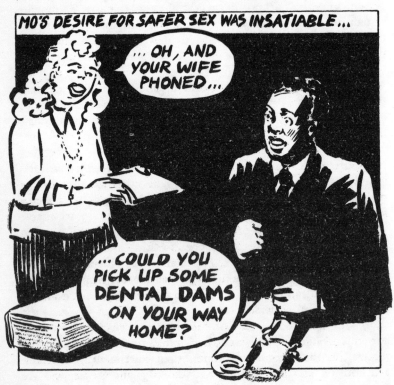

colours, sizes, thicknesses and flavours. Unlike condoms, not many people have heard of them or know where they can be purchased. They are still not widely available, but you can buy them from surgical and dental supply companies, some mail order firms and, increasingly, in shops.

Latex barriers can make oral sex safer as they can be placed over the woman's vulva before cunnilingus and therefore prevent possible HIV transmission through vaginal fluids or blood getting into the active partner's mouth. This works on the same principle as putting a condom on a man's penis during fellatio (see above). They also make rimming (licking or kissing your partner's anus) safer, because placing a latex barrier over the anus prevents HIV, and other infections, from being transmitted.

Other Contraceptives and HIV

The condom is the only contraceptive device that can offer reliable protection against HIV infection. Contraceptive pills do not, because they do nothing to prevent infected semen entering the vagina. The intra-uterine device or coil, diaphragm, cap or contraceptive sponge similarly do not offer protection from HIV, because they do not protect the vaginal walls from possible contact with infected semen. The 'withdrawal' method (when a man removes his penis before ejaculation) is ineffective in preventing HIV transmission just as it is an ineffective contraceptive technique – small amounts of semen are emitted from the penis during sex, even before a man has come.

Natural methods of birth control based on monitoring temperature and cervical mucus have no effect against HIV transmission, neither do female sterilization or vasectomy. They are designed to prevent pregnancy, not infection with a sexually transmitted disease.

The condom for women is a recent development. It is like a thin latex sock which is inserted inside the vagina and fits over the vulva; a kind of cross between the contraceptive cap and a man's condom. It has an inner polyurethane ring which allows it to be inserted and serves to hold it in place over the cervix. There is also an outer ring which fits over the vaginal opening.

As it protects the vagina and cervix from contact with infected semen (and similarly, the penis from contact with infected vaginal fluids), the female condom is thought to be effective against HIV transmission and may be a good alternative for people who are unhappy with condoms for men. At the time of writing it is still not available on the open market, although it is being extensively trialled. Anecdotal reports so far suggest that some women feel that the inner ring of the female condom sitting over the cervix allows deeper penetration than when a male condom is used.

On the other hand, cunnilingus (see above) may be difficult when the female condom is worn, and the noise made by the penis rubbing against the latex may be off-putting for some. A *City Limits* review of the female condom in July 1990 stated that 'Anything approaching sexual athletics and it sounds like a crisp packet being scrumpled up in a pub ashtray.' Whether or not the female condom will turn out to be successful as a safer sex accessory remains to be seen; at this early stage it is thought that women who have difficulties getting men to wear condoms may find it of considerable benefit.

Lubricants and Spermicides

Lubricants play a substantial role in safer sex. They can help to stop the condoms tearing or slipping off during sex by reducing the amount of friction on the rubber. They can also help prevent damage occurring during intercourse to the walls of the vagina or anus due to inadequate lubrication, which in turn can allow HIV and other infections to be absorbed into the body more easily. Thirdly, they can make vaginal or anal penetration and stimulation of the penis and vulva more pleasurable generally.

If you decide to use a lubricant during safer sex, choose a water-based one such as *KY Jelly*, *Duragel* or *Ortho Lubricant*. Do not use oil-based lubricants such as vaseline, hand creams, massage oils or margarine, as they tend to weaken the rubber and make a condom more prone to tearing during sex. Saliva (spit) is also not an effective lubricant. Be careful that you don't confuse water-*based* with water-*soluble* lubricants. Water-soluble lubricants dissolve in water but they still contain oil. Check the packet carefully for details.

You can use lubricants in a number of ways during safer sex. You can rub them into your partner's genitals or all over his or her body. Putting a dab of lubricant on the inside of the tip of a condom helps keep the air out of the condom and stop it from breaking, and also may improve the sensation for a man. Lubricant smeared over the outside of the condom once it has been rolled down a man's erect penis will help reduce friction during vaginal or anal intercourse.

Lubricants are available from chemists, condom manufacturers, and by mail order. The available range is wide, but factors you may like to consider when you choose one are: smell, taste, how long they last, texture, how they feel on your body, how well they lubricate.

Use of a spermicide may also help to make sex safer by inactivating HIV in the vagina and anus. Like lubricants, you can get them from chemists, family planning clinics or mail order companies. Only spermicides containing the chemical *nonoxynol 9, 10* or *11* have been proved to 'kill off' HIV in laboratory tests, but currently most spermicides contain between 1 per cent and 5 per cent of nonoxynol 9; contraceptive foams contain up to 12 per cent. Many condoms are available with spermicide containing nonoxynol 9 already on them; check the packet for details.

It's important to remember that spermicidal creams, gels or foams used on their own are far less effective in safer sex than when used with a condom. It's also important to know that nonoxynol 9 may cause allergic reactions in the vagina or anus, making it easier for HIV to enter the bloodstream. Try testing any spermicide containing nonoxynol 9 on the skin of your wrist first, if you are worried about this. You can always get a different brand of spermicide if you find you do become irritated or sore.

SEX TALK

Safer sex presents us with a series of challenges. It may make us think about the way we feel about our own sexuality, how much sexual experience we have, and how confident we feel about asking for what we want. It may make us aware that we would like more information about sex and handling sexual relationships.

Some people find discussing safer sex easier in ongoing relationships, because they feel closer and more trusting with a long-term partner. For others, it is the feelings of trust and intimacy that confuse the issue: we may be worried that we will upset or offend a long-term partner by talking about safer sex, because it may suggest that the partner is being unfaithful or has a 'promiscuous' background. Studies have shown that sexual partners may not bother with safer sex after a period of time because they have got to know each other better and so do not feel as though they need to worry about HIV. Other couples who have been having unsafe sex for some time may take the attitude that as they have already taken risks, there is no point in bothering with safer sex now.

The trouble with relying on feelings of trust and intimacy to protect you is that it doesn't work. You may feel you have got to know your partner well, but this alone cannot tell you whether you or he or she has HIV infection. And the fact that you may have had regular risky sex before is not a reason to continue taking risks now. Some people have become infected with HIV after just one risky sexual encounter; others have regular risky sex with an infected person and still do not have HIV infection. There is no hard and fast law about exactly how many sexual encounters it takes to pass on the virus. What is certain is that the more times you take risks the greater the likelihood of becoming infected or passing the virus on to someone else.

If you are worried that your partner may think you are suggesting he or she is 'promiscuous' in some way if you raise the subject of safer sex, the information below may help make the discussion more productive. However, it is probably unhelpful to use the term 'promiscuous' at all. As has been said, the number of sexual partners a person has is of less significance in terms of HIV infection than whether he or she is having safer sex with those partners. At the same time, 'promiscuous' is a judgemental term which can offend and alienate; it also means very different things to different people. Most of us would find it difficult to decide how many sexual partners a person needs to have to be labelled promiscuous; for many of us, a promiscuous person may just mean someone who has more sexual partners than we do.

In some relationships there is a threat of violence, abuse, sexual assault or rape. These are problems women (and some men) have been faced with for years, and they may make discussion of safer sex an impossibility. Similarly, fears that talking about safer sex may encourage your partner to seek sex with someone else or to leave you altogether are very real deterrents for many people, particularly if they are emotionally or economically dependent on their partner. Again, women are generally hardest hit by these worries, and there is no simple answer to them. If you are in a situation where you risk mental or physical abuse or are scared about being left by your partner, you are likely to need professional support and advice. In the Directory at the back of this book there is a list of organisations which may be able to help you.

Safer sex cannot be put in a neat little box and kept separate from the rest of our lives. Who we are and how we live affects our ability to think about, plan and negotiate safer sex. Stress from other factors in our lives such as fatigue, family and workplace problems, lack of exercise, poor health and lack of money all have an impact upon our sexual activity.

If you have stressful situations to deal with you may well need the help and support of other people. Just being aware of what may get in the way of safer sex is a good start. The next step is thinking about and practising the basic guidelines to safer sexual negotiation.

Making a Start

It helps to have an atmosphere in which you can be as relaxed and calm as possible to talk about safer sex with your partner. Shouting out your insistence on using condoms or having non-penetrative sex to a new partner on a disco dance-floor could be unproductive as well as embarrassing. The most important thing is to be somewhere peaceful enough to talk comfortably and without interruption. It may also be easier to find somewhere neutral to talk, so that neither of you feels pressurised - your bedroom or your partner's bedroom may not necessarily be this place. You will need to think about what is possible and what feels right for you.

Safer sex may take quite a lot of time to talk about, particularly if it is the first time you have raised it with anybody. There is no universal rule about when to bring it up; it will depend on how ready you feel and how you think the subject will be received. It is probably best not to discuss safer sex when you or your partner are feeling tired, depressed, angry or ill. It is also best not to wait until the very last minute, when you are about to have sex and are both feeling very aroused - that situation is unlikely to allow you to think clearly enough to say what you want to say. You may feel that it would be a shame to spoil the passion of the moment by talking about safety, and not bother.

Safer sex requires time, space, energy and commitment. If you rush both talking about and doing it, you may find you are missing out.

Drugs and alcohol might help you to relax with a new partner, but they could make it more difficult for you to decide to stay safe. If your judgement is affected, you might end up ignoring the risks and having risky sex. One way to deal with this is by deciding your limit beforehand and sticking with it. If you know you are likely to be in a situation which could lead to sex, try to keep a clear head. This does not mean you have to stick to alcohol-free lager or orange juice, unless you want to. It does mean that you have to pace yourself, or plan ahead so that any discussion about safer sex takes place before drinking or drug-taking does.

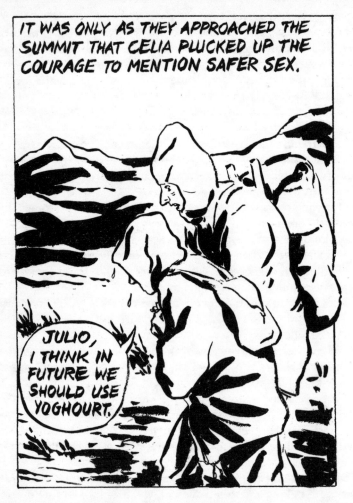

Drugs and alcohol are not just a potential danger in sexual negotiation; they also affect your health. If you are a person with HIV, the effects of regular drug or alcohol use could be more serious. They could weaken your immune system further and make you more vulnerable to other infections (see Chapters 5 and 7).

Talking about the kind of sex you enjoy may be difficult. You may not know what turns you on, or you may find the subject of sex too embarrassing to mention. Part of the problem may be the sexual language that is available to us. Some words can seem too clinical, vague, or crude for us to use. Only you can decide what terms you feel comfortable with, and talking to your partner about this will make it easier to avoid embarrassment and misunderstanding. Why not try writing down some of the words you both know for parts of the body and sexual activities and agreeing on those you feel happy with? Some couples develop their own private languages for different ways of having sex, and this need not be an uncomfortable exercise: it could be fun.

Effective sexual communication depends on being able to express what you want to say clearly and simply. Partners do not necessarily know what we want without being told, and getting straightforward messages can dispense with a lot of frustrating guesswork on both sides. There is no reason why talking about sex should mean that imagination and sensitivity are sacrificed along the way – in fact, the opposite. If you know what you and your partner want there is more space for creative and pleasurable sex than if you are literally groping in the dark.

Safer sexual negotiation is likely to involve knowing and using assertive techniques, because once you are clear what you want, you may need to repeat the message several times and deal with a series of arguments aimed at putting you off the idea. It also involves listening skills, because you need to hear and understand what your partner is saying and why he or she feels like that.

Above all, it helps to remember that talking about safer sex needn't be a grim and gloomy discussion; it could be very amusing! If you can have a laugh with your partner, the situation can become a lot easier to manage. If you are able to make safer sex sound like fun, it is more likely to *be* fun.

Safer sex involves balancing respect for your partner with respect for yourself. It may be possible to find a compromise that will make you both happy, or it may not. If it is not, and if despite all your assertiveness, persuasion or even pleading your partner refuses to budge on the matter, you are faced with a big question. That is: how long can you spend and how high a price are you prepared to pay for staying in a relationship where safer sex is not negotiable?

6

THE HIV ANTIBODY TEST

When American scientists were given licences by the US Department of Health in 1984 to develop a blood test for HIV infection, they were aware of the limitations of such a test. No simple blood test could be used to diagnose AIDS itself, since by definition AIDS is a complex medical condition rather than (like HIV) a viral infection. Neither, however, was it feasible to produce a test which would detect HIV infection, since to do so would have been far too laborious and time-consuming. Part of the problem is that, even when a person with HIV is at a particularly infectious stage (for example, just after he or she has become HIV positive) there is very little virus circulating in the bloodstream. This makes it difficult for a test to pick up the presence of HIV.

It was clear that tests would have to rely on the presence of *antibodies* to the virus as a marker for infection. In the majority of people with HIV, antibodies develop within three to six months from the date of infection. They are generally present in the blood in sufficient quantity to be fairly easy to detect. Thus, when in March 1985 a commercially available test had finally been developed in the US, it was neither a test for AIDS nor for HIV infection, but a test for antibodies; the HIV antibody test.

HOW THE HIV ANTIBODY TEST WORKS

The most widely available HIV antibody test is called the ELISA test; or *enzyme-linked immunosorbent assay*. A positive result is indicated by a colour change. If no change takes place, there are no antibodies in the sample.

If there are HIV antibodies, the test result is said to be *positive*. If not, the result is *negative*. Positive test results are confirmed with a *Western blot test*, which uses a different technique.

The Western blot test is more complicated and more accurate than the ELISA test. It is capable of detecting a range of different antibodies that may be produced in response to HIV infection, which the ELISA test is unable to do. The Western blot technique works by separating different proteins of HIV, putting them in a liquid gel and exposing them to an electric current. The proteins form themselves into a column, with the lighter and faster-moving proteins at one end and the heavier, slower ones at the other. The 'column' of proteins is moved onto strips of nitrocellulose gel and exposed to a blood sample. If the sample contains antibodies these will bind to the proteins on the strips. Radioactive chemicals, which will stick to the antibodies if they are present, are then added. If there are HIV antibodies in the blood sample, the radioactive chemicals will cause the viral proteins to show up on the photographic sheet. If there are no antibodies, the chemicals have nothing to stick to, so there will be no image of the viral proteins.

THE ACCURACY OF HIV ANTIBODY TESTS

The ELISA antibody test that is currently used is said to have a *sensitivity* of around 97 per cent and a *specificity* of about 99 per cent. These terms may sound confusing at first, but they simply refer to the probability that the test will detect HIV antibodies in the blood when they *are* present and not mistakenly indicate their presence when they are *not* present. A test that is 100 per cent sensitive, therefore, will always give a positive result when there *are* HIV antibodies in the blood, and a test that is 100 per cent specific will always give a negative result when there are no HIV antibodies in the blood.

In an ideal world, the ELISA test would be 100 per cent sensitive and 100 per cent specific. As it is, the 99 per cent specificity rate means that one out of every 100 blood samples taken could be falsely identified as positive for HIV antibodies. Being given a positive antibody test result can be a traumatic experience, as is discussed later in this chapter, so double-checking a positive result with the Western blot test is very important (doctors will do this as a matter of course).

There is another reason, however, why HIV antibody testing will never be absolutely accurate. A person with HIV does not usually develop antibodies to the virus straightaway. As mentioned above, on average this takes about three months to happen, although occasionally it takes less or more time than this (in a very few cases people with HIV are reported never to have developed HIV antibodies, their HIV status being discovered only when they develop AIDS-related symptoms). The time span between infection with HIV and development of antibodies is called the 'window of infection' period, and if a person with HIV takes the antibody test during that period, he or she will receive a negative test result even though HIV positive, because no antibodies to the virus will have had time to develop.

For this reason, if you decide to take the HIV antibody test it is always a good idea to wait until at least three months have gone by since the date when you think you may have been infected. (It is also a good idea to read the rest of this chapter before you make any decision about taking the test.)

TESTING DEVELOPMENTS

Although the most widely available test for infection is the HIV antibody test (i.e. the ELISA), scientific advances over the past few years suggest that HIV antigen testing may play a more prominent role in the future. (An antigen is any foreign substance in the body, so an HIV antigen is simply a particle of HIV.)

HIV antigen testing has the advantage of detecting the virus in people who have only recently become infected with HIV, who would therefore receive a negative antibody test result because their bodies have not yet produced antibodies to the virus.

Antigen testing is problematic, however. While it is true that at the time of infection (and before the body has had a chance to produce antibodies) viral antigen will be present in the body in detectable quantity, as soon as antibodies develop, viral antigen diminishes. People with HIV who are asymptomatic (have no symptoms of illness) tend to have low levels of viral antigen, whereas people with HIV-related immune deficiency generally have higher antigen levels. This makes antigen testing extremely difficult for the vast majority of asymptomatic people with HIV. In general, antigen testing techniques are currently considered too time-consuming, difficult and expensive to replace antibody testing as a means of detecting HIV infection.

Recently, researchers have examined the possibilities of testing samples of urine and saliva instead of blood for HIV antibodies. Studies have shown levels of sensitivity and specificity that compare well to those available from HIV antibody testing of blood samples. The advantages of this are that such testing would be non-invasive; in other words it would not involve inserting a needle into someone's arm to draw blood.

There are clear advantages to taking samples of urine and saliva in terms of the ease and simplicity of administering the tests. However, the development of saliva and urine testing kits suggest that in the near future it may well become possible for individuals to buy these off the shelf for their own private use. It is important to sound a strong note of warning about this. As stated later in this chapter, it is crucial that HIV antibody testing is always accompanied by pre- and post-test counselling. People need to think about the kind of effect taking the test might have on their lives before they can make an informed decision about whether or not to go ahead with it. Whether the result is HIV negative or positive, it is likely that they would need further information and support.

WHERE IS THE TEST AVAILABLE?

In Britain, HIV antibody tests are available free from genito-urinary (GU) clinics (also called sexually transmitted disease or STD clinics), general practitioners, and some private health clinics.

The two most important issues to consider when you are thinking about where to take the HIV antibody test are whether your test result will be kept confidential (some of the reasons for this are discussed below) and whether adequate counselling will be provided for you before and after taking the test.

Pre- and post-test counselling are very important because they help you to think about why you want to know your HIV antibody status and how it might feel if you had a positive test result. If you are HIV positive, you may well need advice and support to deal with the news, as well as with any changes in your life you may want to make. If your test result is negative, information about how to avoid HIV infection may well be necessary. So counselling can serve a number of important functions: it helps you to focus upon whether or not to take the test, provides information about staying safe and protecting other people, and gives support and help if you have a positive test result.

It may well be best to go to a National Health Service STD or GU clinic if you are considering taking the HIV antibody test, because these have the best safeguards for protecting confidentiality. Whereas breach of confidence is unlawful in any aspect of medical care, at GU and STD clinics there is an additional law (the VD Act) which makes it illegal for the clinic to let anyone else know that a person has taken the HIV antibody test, or what the result was, unless that person has specifically agreed to this. Most clinics also offer pre- and post-test counselling, although you may wish to check this first.

If you choose to go to a GU or STD clinic for the test, it is possible that the doctor you deal with will want to notify your GP of your test result. Whether or not you are happy for this to happen will depend on your circumstances. If you have HIV illness, it may well be advisable for your GP to know so that any future infections can be diagnosed and treated as promptly as possible.

However, if you have HIV but no symptoms of illness you may need to think very carefully about whether or not your GP should know your HIV antibody status. If you trust your GP to keep the information confidential, you may be happy for him or her to know. However, if you have any concerns that he or she might pass the information to others against your wishes, the best advice is not to allow the clinic to inform your GP. Also be aware that GPs are legally bound to pass on information to insurance advisers about patients' HIV antibody status.

Although the doctor you deal with at the clinic should respect your wishes should you not want your GP informed, there are other ways of avoiding potential difficulties with this. You do not need to give your real name to the clinic, for example (it is however a good idea to make sure you provide an address where the clinic doctor can reach you if necessary). Alternatively, before you agree to take the test you could ask the clinic doctor whether he or she wants to tell your GP about your test result. If the answer is yes, you can always go to another clinic if you still want to take the test; you are not obliged to go to the clinic in your area. It may help to check that staff understand the importance of confidentiality if you have any doubts about this.

In general there is little to be gained from going to your GP for the HIV antibody test. Although some GPs are very responsible about maintaining confidentiality, others are not. It is also possible that you will not be offered counselling before the test, or afterwards if you do take it. Similarly, private clinics are not likely to be a better bet than an NHS clinic. They charge for a service which is provided elsewhere for free, and you cannot always be certain either that the test result will be kept confidential or that counselling will be available (some clinics provide this, but only at extra cost).

THINKING ABOUT TAKING THE TEST

The test is conducted by taking a small sample of blood from a vein in your arm. The blood sample will then be sent with others to different national testing centres, so receiving your test result may take anything from one to three weeks. If you receive a positive test result it means that you have HIV infection and will probably always be infectious to other people. If you receive a negative test result it means that you do not have HIV infection or that you have not yet developed the antibodies – so be careful not to take the test before antibodies to HIV have had a chance to develop. Positive test results are double-checked with the Western blot technique, as described above.

Sometimes it is possible to get 'same day' testing at a clinic. This might help if you feel you want to get the test over and done with, but be careful. It's very important to make sure that you have had enough time to think the matter through carefully. One day might not be enough.

There are all kinds of reasons for taking the HIV antibody test, and as many for avoiding it. Before you make a decision about whether to take the test or not, you may find this section of the book helpful in weighing up the pros and cons. Whatever your decision, it must be yours alone. Do not let anyone rush you into taking the test, or try to make up your mind for you. You may want to read further literature about testing, or contact an organisation that can give you further help and advice on this issue; see the Directory at the back of this book for details.

Your feelings about whether or not to take the HIV antibody test can be flexible – deciding that it is inappropriate now does not mean that you may not change your mind in the future.

Some Reasons for Taking the Test

- For some people the issue may not be *whether* to take the test, but *when*. This is because although there is still no cure for HIV infection, new drugs to treat or delay illness in people with HIV are continually being researched and trialled. As time goes on it is increasingly likely that people who are diagnosed early with HIV infection will be able to avoid serious illness through careful medical monitoring (regular check-ups and blood tests) and the use of effective preventive therapies. This is sometimes called 'early intervention'. Although we are not yet at a stage where available drugs are considered to be entirely effective in preventing HIV illness, the regular check-ups and blood tests a doctor could provide might make it worth taking the test for a person who thinks he or she is likely to get a positive result.

Similarly, if you are ill and the chances are high that the illness is HIV-related, taking the test may help your doctor to diagnose and treat you more quickly.

- If you feel that you have been at risk of HIV infection, knowing for sure that you are HIV positive could mean that you are able to concentrate on looking after your health and making changes to the way you live, in order to reduce the risk of getting ill (Chapter 7 looks at this in detail).

- If you are in a stable relationship where you or your partner have possibly been exposed to HIV infection and are worried about whether or not to practise safer sex, taking the HIV antibody test may help you to decide on appropriate sexual activities. You and your partner may decide to take the test together. If you test HIV negative, remember that you will not be able to have unsafe sex with your partner unless you know he or she is also HIV negative.

 It is worth thinking this option through carefully, however. If you and your partner are HIV negative, the only way to stay negative is for both of you to avoid risky sex (or risky drug use) with other people. If the relationship ends, then you have no guarantee that your next sexual partner will be HIV negative. Another point to consider is the impact upon your relationship of a situation where one of you is HIV negative and the other HIV positive.

- If you are very anxious and concerned about your HIV antibody status, even though you are not really sure that you have put yourself at risk, taking the test may help to put your fears to rest. Some people may become so worried about whether or not they have HIV infection that taking the test seems to offer reassurance, even with the risk of a positive result.

 Again, you might want to think carefully about this. If you received a positive test result, how would that feel? If the test result were negative, would that put an end to your worries? Some people take the HIV antibody test repeatedly, even if they keep getting a negative result. This may be due to worries about sexuality, difficulties with a sexual relationship, or a range of other reasons. If you think that you might find it hard to accept a negative test result, it is possible that you may have other worries on your mind that a counsellor could help you to talk through, but which a test on its own might not solve.

- If you have been practising unsafe sex or drug use, taking the test *may* encourage you to change your behaviour. If you are HIV negative, you will want to stay that way, and if you are HIV positive you will want to think about not passing the virus on to other people. (However, it is important to remember that you don't need to know your HIV antibody status in order to practise safer behaviour; you might want to think about staying safe in any case.)

- Women who feel they may have HIV infection and who want to have a baby could find that knowing their HIV antibody status helps to clarify the decision about whether to get pregnant or not, or whether or not to continue a pregnancy. It now appears that for women with HIV but no symptoms of illness the chance of passing the virus to the baby before birth is around one in five. So even if you have a positive test result you may still wish to have a baby (see Chapter 4 for further information).

  If you take the test in order to make a decision about getting pregnant in the future, your partner will also need to be tested. If you plan to try insemination through a donor clinic, the sperm donated is always tested for HIV antibodies (see Chapter 4). However, if you want to make your own private arrangements, remember to make sure that the donor has been tested also.

- Similarly, women who think they may have HIV and are breastfeeding their baby might find that taking the test will help them to decide whether to continue breastfeeding (in a few reported cases, HIV has been transmitted to babies from the mother through breastmilk).

  Mothers who are uncertain whether to have their babies immunised with the BCG vaccine for tuberculosis, which is harmful to people with immune deficiency, might find that taking the HIV antibody test will clarify the situation (Chapter 7 gives more information on vaccination and HIV, but it is always worth asking your doctor for the latest information).

  If the mother is HIV negative, then her baby will also be negative. If the mother is positive, then she may wish to wait until her baby is old enough to be given an HIV antibody test before making a decision about vaccination.

- If travel requires you to be vaccinated or immunised with a live attenuated virus, you might want to find out your HIV antibody status and get the latest information about which vaccines are safe.

- If you have to go to a country where HIV tests for foreign residents are compulsory, it may well be better to take the test in Britain, if you think it is likely to be positive. More information is given about international testing policy in Chapter 9.

Some Reasons for Not Taking the Test

- Many people take the test in the hope that it will provide reassurance about their HIV antibody status. However, if the test result is positive the opposite may be the case. Common reactions to a positive test result include shock, anger, confusion, depression and acute anxiety. Some people find that the shock may cause them to feel numb and withdrawn from others temporarily, while others have felt desperate and suicidal. This range of responses to being HIV positive is one of the reasons why pre- and post-test counselling are so important.

  Again, the first question to ask yourself is 'How would I feel if the test result was positive?' This is by no means easy to answer, so take all the time you need to consider this. The decision to test or not to test is far too important to rush. You may feel that you will be able to handle your reactions if you are HIV positive, but if after thinking it through you are still unsure whether or not you could cope with a positive result, it might be best to wait before taking the test.

- A test result is no substitute for safer behaviour. If you are HIV negative you will want to stay that way, and if you are HIV positive you will want to avoid infecting sexual partners or putting yourself at risk of sexual infections through unsafe sex.

  If you decide to take the test, and receive a negative result, you may find that you are tempted to take risks because of a false sense of security. A negative test result today will not keep you safe from HIV infection for the rest of your life, unless you practise safer behaviour. If you think that the relief of knowing you are HIV negative may encourage you to have unsafe sex or share needles to inject drugs, it might be best to avoid taking the test.

- Despite all the information available on HIV, many people still believe that it is transmitted through casual social contact, and are afraid of people with HIV infection. In addition to fear, they may have prejudiced views about people with HIV (such as gay men, injecting drug users, or people they see as 'promiscuous') being responsible for spreading the virus, or having 'only themselves to blame' for getting infected.

  Having a positive test result could be a shock, and the urge to get support and help from your friends and family may be very strong. However, if you decide to take the test you will need to think very carefully about whom (if anyone) you would want to tell about receiving a positive result. Some people have found that their friends, relatives or lover(s) have been unable to cope with the knowledge that they have HIV, and have rejected or isolated them. Others have found that the test result was not kept confidential by people they trusted with the information.

Feeling secure that you have reliable support from people who are caring and sensitive to your needs and aware of the significance of confidentiality is very important. If you are unsure that you can rely on receiving such support, it may be best not to take the test, or to delay taking it until you are confident that the support you need is available.

- Sometimes the idea of taking the test is served up to us in media coverage of HIV issues as a socially responsible move. We may continually come across stories about well-known people who took the test because they wanted to be responsible to a current sexual partner, or to future partners. This suggests that taking the HIV antibody test on its own can prevent HIV transmission. Obviously this is not so. Knowing your HIV antibody status is of little relevance if you do not try to stay safe or protect other people from infection. And you do not need to take the test in order to do that.

- People with HIV may experience severe discrimination in the areas of housing, education, employment, insurance and travel. Brief information about the range of discrimination related to HIV antibody status is given in the following section. Chapter 7 offers practical advice for people who are HIV positive on ways of dealing with discrimination in different settings.

HIV AND DISCRIMINATION

Life Assurance
There are two key reasons why a person might consider life assurance – by itself, to protect his or her partner and others who may be dependent in the case of death; or in association with a mortgage upon a property. However, the HIV epidemic has made life assurance companies extremely cautious about the clients they will insure. Unfortunately, assurance companies continue to see clients in terms of 'high-risk groups' rather than considering unsafe behaviour as the element that confers risk. They do not, for example, appear to recognise that gay men who practise safer sex are at considerably lower risk of HIV infection than, say, heterosexual men who do not.

Companies are legally entitled to refuse to insure whomever they wish, and do not need to provide reasons for the decision. A company will definitely refuse to offer you life assurance if you have HIV; or if you refuse to take the HIV antibody test when asked by the company; or if you do not give consent either to a medical examination or for your doctor to be approached for a medical report.

Furthermore, it is quite probable that a company will refuse you assurance (or else impose special terms upon it) for a range of other reasons. For example, if you are gay (or if the company thinks that you are) you may well be refused life assurance, or offered it at a much higher premium. If you have had an HIV antibody test (even if the result was negative), if you are a person with haemophilia, an injecting drug user, or a single man sharing accommodation with another single man, then a life assurance company may refuse to provide cover. Similarly, if the company knows or suspects you to have had previous sexually transmitted diseases, to have a history of injecting drug use or haemophilia, or to have previously applied unsuccessfully for life assurance elsewhere, then you may be regarded as too great a risk to take on.

If you are thinking of applying for life assurance (or a mortgage which involves assurance cover) and think there is a chance that you may be refused, it is a good idea to get further advice and information. If you have HIV infection there is little point in trying to obtain ordinary life assurance (because you will not be able to get it), but you may well be able to get a mortgage; see *Life Assurance and Mortgages* in Chapter 7. Some of the organisations listed in the Directory at the back of this book can provide literature giving further information and usually have advisers to talk you through the issues.

HIV and Employment

Sensible policy guidelines and HIV education programmes are excellent ways of preventing fear and stigma about HIV antibody status in the workplace. Despite this, people with HIV, or who are suspected of having HIV, continue to experience harassment, abuse and discrimination from employers and colleagues. Gay men and people with haemophilia are particularly at risk of this, because of the long-standing associations between homosexuality, haemophilia and HIV.

In March 1986, guidelines on HIV in the workplace were issued jointly by the Department of Employment and the Health and Safety Executive, and sent to every employer in Britain. The *AIDS and the Workplace* booklet states that the risk of HIV transmission in the workplace is negligible, even for employees in health care services. It also says that dismissing people with HIV, purely on the grounds that other employees want this, would 'in many cases expose the employer to a claim for unfair dismissal'.

Unfortunately, it's not quite as simple as that. If you feel that you have been unfairly dismissed from your job, be aware that you need to have been employed with a company for two years before you can take your case to an industrial tribunal. Even then, there is no guarantee that you will get your job back.

Although trade unions and voluntary organisations have become involved in HIV and employment matters and have produced policy guidelines and information for employers about HIV transmission, testing, counselling and support, the workplace is still an area where approaches to HIV and AIDS vary enormously. Some organisations have ensured that adequate information and training on HIV and AIDS are made available to all employees. Others have dismissed workers with HIV, or insisted that all job applicants take an HIV antibody test (and turned away any who refuse to take the test, or who test HIV positive).

For this reason, if you have HIV infection, it is very important to think carefully about keeping the information confidential (this issue is looked at in more depth in Chapter 7). If you are applying for a job with a company which insists that its new employees take an HIV antibody test, you will again need to think carefully about your options. Even though HIV is not transmitted through ordinary social contact, employers are not prevented by law from introducing HIV antibody tests for new employees.

However, employers who try to force current employees to take the test are acting outside their rights. If your employer says that the test is compulsory, and you refuse to take it, this could be equivalent to employer's breach of contract. In this case you would be entitled to hand in your notice and claim constructive dismissal.

These are issues which require more detailed discussion than this book can provide. You need to think carefully and have the best information available if you feel you are being discriminated against by your employer with regard to your actual or suspected HIV antibody status. Chapter 7 may provide some useful further reading, and organisations listed in the Directory at the back of this book can offer you further help and advice.

Travel

People with HIV may face difficulties if they wish to live, work or study abroad, because some countries have decided to impose compulsory HIV antibody tests on foreigners applying for visas, study or work permits. A person with a positive test result is likely to be refused access to the country in question. In other cases, people judged to be 'at high risk of HIV' have been compulsorily tested upon arrival or during their stay in a country, and deported if found to be HIV positive.

Countries involved in such measures are wide-ranging; they exist on every continent. However, one of the difficulties of getting up-to-date information on the situation in any particular country is that travel restrictions may operate on an unofficial level, even if the country has no formal policy to discriminate. Another problem is that there is no consistent global picture; trends are constantly changing, so that HIV antibody testing for some or all categories of foreign visitor may be viewed as unnecessary one month and compulsory the next.

If you are planning to go abroad for any reason you need to know the likelihood of being forced to take the HIV antibody test in order to get a travel visa. It may help to contact organisations which can give you further advice and information, some of which are listed in the Directory at the back of this book. In some situations, such as work or study abroad, you may have little choice in the matter. It is important to remember, however, that if you do decide to take the test in order to be able to travel, it may very well have a much greater effect on your life than you had anticipated. You will also have little control over who has access to information about your test result.

Imposing immigration restrictions upon foreign visitors with HIV is unlikely to succeed as a means of limiting the spread of the epidemic. Closed borders will never have any effect upon a virus which can now be found throughout the world, although they may have a serious impact upon the international co-operation necessary to provide adequate research, treatment, education and counselling programmes globally.

Housing

In many of Britain's large towns and cities, finding appropriate, affordable housing is already a considerable difficulty even for people who are HIV negative and without health problems. For people with HIV these difficulties may be exacerbated by the ignorance and prejudice of others. While in some areas housing associations and authorities have developed sensitive and carefully considered accommodation policies on the issues of HIV and AIDS, in other areas people with HIV have been refused accommodation or evicted from rented premises by discriminatory landlords. Harassment and violence may also be experienced at the hands of hostile neighbours who continue to entertain the myth that HIV can be easily transmitted, and that those with HIV infection do not deserve decent living conditions.

This book cannot give the kind of detailed advice you will require if you are a person with HIV (or who is presumed to have HIV) experiencing harassment or discrimination in connection with your housing needs. Chapter 7 outlines some of the options that may be available to you. It is sensible to get advice from organisations working in housing and HIV (see the Directory at the back of this book) before you disclose your antibody status to anyone; they may also be able to give you information about what is available in your area and where and how to obtain legal support if you need it.

TESTING POLICY

Testing blood samples for HIV antibodies has a number of different uses. It can be used to protect a country's supply of donated blood, blood products and internal organs, or as a voluntary diagnostic tool for individuals who may be concerned about their HIV antibody status. This section looks at two further uses of the HIV antibody test: compulsory testing, which may involve the enforcement of discriminatory measures against people with HIV, and anonymous testing, where the test is used as a means of gaining up-to-date information about the prevalence of HIV infection throughout a population.

Compulsory Testing

Ever since HIV was identified in 1983 there have been some unsuccessful calls for the introduction of compulsory HIV antibody testing. Introducing compulsory testing would mean that individuals could be tested for HIV antibodies without their consent and could be forced to comply by law.

There are all sorts of reasons why implementing a programme of compulsory testing, either for selected groups or entire populations, could well turn into an expensive disaster. To begin with, the discrimination levelled at people with a positive antibody test result makes forcing individuals to take the test highly unethical.

Secondly, it is extremely doubtful that a compulsory testing programme would yield any useful information. A testing programme of this sort would only identify people who are HIV negative *today*; it would offer no guarantee that the same people would still be HIV negative in a few weeks' or months' time. Without effective education about safer behaviour, HIV antibody testing is worth little.

Similarly, due to the 'window of infection' period described above, compulsory testing would be open to considerable inaccuracy: people recently infected with HIV who had not yet developed antibodies would be wrongly identified as HIV negative. There is also the fact that antibody tests for HIV are not 100 per cent effective; their margin of error would have serious implications for mass compulsory testing.

Coercion tends to generate fear and hostility, which do not create fertile ground for HIV prevention work. Compulsory testing might reinforce the misconceptions that have dogged HIV education since it began: that the virus is casually transmitted, and that those with HIV should be avoided at all costs. In such an atmosphere, it is highly likely that people with HIV would stay away from the medical, counselling and social services set up to help them. Those who perceive themselves as at risk of HIV infection would be unwilling to seek information and advice. In other words, the HIV epidemic could be forced underground, at considerable cost to the individual and to the State.

In 1987, the House of Commons Social Services Committee ruled out compulsory HIV antibody testing as an effective HIV prevention measure in Britain. Nevertheless, we cannot afford to be complacent about this. Maintaining infection control procedures costs money, but then so does HIV antibody testing. The difference is that the first has been shown to be a successful HIV prevention measure; the second has not.

Anonymous Testing

In late 1988, the British Government announced that a programme of anonymous testing would be introduced. Anonymous testing is a process by which blood samples taken from individuals for a range of clinically necessary tests are also later tested for HIV antibodies.

After the tests for other infections are performed, all identifying information is removed from the blood sample, although information such as the sex of the donor and (if known) the way HIV infection occurred may be recorded. When the removal of identifying information has made it impossible to trace the original donor, the blood may be tested for HIV antibodies.

This process is called 'anonymous screening', because the doctor performing the test will have no idea to whom the blood belongs. This also means that information about a person's antibody status cannot be passed on to other people. The person whose blood it is will not be given the result of the HIV antibody test, because the blood sample cannot be traced to him or her.

In January 1990, the anonymous screening programme was launched in Britain on a massive scale, involving pregnant women attending antenatal clinics, injecting drug users, and people visiting GU clinics. The programme's launch was preceded by a year of anonymous testing for HIV antibodies among 114,515 babies from whom blood samples had been routinely collected for other purposes. It is anticipated that the anonymous testing programme currently underway will also later extend to involve hospital outpatients.

People attending clinics where anonymous screening of blood samples is taking place should be given information about the programme so that they are clear how it works, and that they understand that their blood sample may be tested. They can refuse to allow their blood to be anonymously tested for HIV antibodies, although their *explicit* consent to anonymous testing is not necessary. In other words, if you are attending a GU or antenatal clinic for tests unrelated to HIV and are made aware that your blood may be tested anonymously for HIV antibodies, you can refuse to allow this. If you do not refuse, tacit consent will be assumed.

It is important that the advantages and disadvantages of anonymous screening are clear. At present the most accurate picture of levels of HIV infection and AIDS is dependent upon a voluntary and confidential reporting system. Data is supplied from several sources – such as general practitioners, GU clinics and blood transfusion services – to the Communicable Diseases Surveillance Centre (CDSC) in Colindale, North London, and the Communicable Diseases (Scotland) Unit (CD(S)U). (What is provided are numbers of cases of HIV and AIDS rather than identifying information about individuals.) The Public Health Laboratory Service (PHLS) compiles regular up-to-date records of the number of people with HIV and AIDS in Britain, and circulates these in the form of monthly reports to people working in the field. The Department of Health also provides monthly press releases updating journalists and the general public on HIV and AIDS statistics.

One of the problems with relying on this system for up-to-date HIV figures is that many people with HIV infection are unlikely to know that they have the virus. They may see no reason for taking an HIV antibody test, and therefore will not be included in official statistics, or they may be put off taking the test for other reasons, such as possible discrimination. Anonymous screening is therefore seen as the method of providing the most accurate idea of how HIV has affected different social groups, and how it relates to factors such as age, sex, sexual orientation and a previous history of other sexually transmitted diseases.

Those in favour of it argue that, by providing a better understanding of the spread of HIV, anonymous testing will make possible a more realistic assessment of future resource allocation and planning of HIV and AIDS services. It may also allow more effective and appropriate targetting of public education and health promotion programmes about HIV.

Those who disagree with the anonymous testing programme may do so on a number of different grounds. Some people feel that there is an ethical problem about implementing a programme where people may be tested for HIV antibodies but cannot receive the test results. Information about HIV antibody status may be crucial to an individual in a range of ways: to gain better medical care and treatment, to assess the viability of continuing with pregnancy or getting pregnant, to make decisions about assurance applications, and so on.

It is argued that the anonymous testing programme will not provide helpful information for adequate resourcing and planning of future health care, social services and education programmes on HIV infection. Although current HIV figures are not comprehensive, predictions of the future spread of HIV and development of AIDS in Britain have been available for several years. This has not, however, necessarily meant that health and social services have automatically received the funding they have asked for to cope with the growing number of people with HIV illness for whom they care. It appears increasingly likely that information about safe behaviour will be necessary for people of all ages, cultural backgrounds and sexualities as the epidemic progresses, so anonymous testing may be of limited relevance to the planning of HIV education.

Another argument against the anonymous testing programme is that, as for compulsory testing, it may generate little useful data. In the pilot study among babies in 1989, levels of HIV infection found among the babies' blood samples were very low – around one infected sample in every 2,000 in the inner London area and under one in 20,000 outside London. This type of testing may also dissuade people from seeking antenatal care or other sorts of medical help, while others may feel uncertain about the practical aspects of the way the programme is implemented.

Despite the division of views about anonymous testing, it is clear that a voluntary testing programme cannot be relied upon to provide a comprehensive picture of HIV infection and AIDS in Britain. While discrimination against people with HIV and AIDS remains a possibility, it is likely that those who think they may have HIV infection will be unwilling to take the HIV antibody test, and that voluntary testing will provide only incomplete data about the spread of HIV.

Discrimination is not only unethical and unnecessary, it is also extremely unhelpful in terms of our understanding of the prevalence of HIV and AIDS. So far much of what we know about HIV and AIDS has been learned because HIV-positive people have given their time, energy and commitment to making more information available. While protection from discrimination is not guaranteed, the continued input and involvement of people with HIV in research, treatment and counselling programmes will remain uncertain.

7

LIVING WITH HIV AND AIDS

Having HIV made me clean up, stop using drugs. I saw that as a quick way to kill myself. I went from being a heavy drug user to wanting to live.

Many people believe that if you have HIV, you don't have an open-ended future. But I feel alive. I try not to create limitations for myself. I want to make my own open-ended future.

In 1990, the Terrence Higgins Trust produced a video for young people about HIV and AIDS, bringing together a group of students (aged 19 to 30) and three people with HIV illness to talk about their experiences. The statements above were recorded during a discussion about living with HIV infection; most of the students claimed to find it an informative but shocking exercise. Prior to taking part in the video, many of them had not recognised that people with HIV can have sexual relationships, work, go out for the evening and enjoy themselves in the same way as people who are HIV negative. Many participants said that they had learned more from being able to talk directly to people with HIV than from any posters, leaflets and television advertisements they had seen on the subject.

Unfortunately, the vast majority of people in Britain do not (or think they do not) know anybody with HIV. Perhaps if more people were prepared to learn directly from the experiences of those with HIV, and could put human faces to what is often seen purely in statistical terms, much of the prejudice and discrimination attached to this viral condition might be removed. As it is, being able to live well with HIV infection remains a question of handling not only the possibility of future illness, but also the possibility of rejection and stigmatisation by others.

Living with HIV is also affected by social, financial and domestic arrangements. Getting out and about and meeting friends depends on having the friends, and the money, to do so. Establishing a worthwhile and rewarding routine at work depends on being able to keep working, or having a job to begin with. Inadequate housing, poverty, loneliness, rejection by family, lover and friends are all factors which can make life much tougher for someone who is HIV positive. This chapter looks at basic self-help techniques for positive living and provides information about getting help and advice to deal with the practical problems HIV infection often poses.

There is enough information on living with HIV to fill entire books; one chapter cannot cover it all. However, if you want to read further on the subject some useful publications are listed in the Directory at the back of this book. Chapter 8 of this book deals with caring for a person with HIV and related illness, but much of the information given in this chapter will also be relevant to carers.

GETTING A DIAGNOSIS OF HIV INFECTION OR AIDS

People with HIV sometimes talk about 'death by duvet'. This is what happens when a person who has recently received an AIDS diagnosis slides into a state of depression, goes home, pulls the duvet over his or her head and lies there quietly, waiting for death.

Fortunately, the onset of extreme boredom with staying in bed is a far more likely outcome of this activity. However, the depression and despair that prompt a desire to give up and wait for the worst to happen are understandable reactions when faced with a life-threatening infection. If you have recently been given a positive HIV antibody test or AIDS diagnosis, you may well find that your response to the news is completely unpredictable. Shock, anger and confusion are just some of the feelings you may be experiencing.

DEALING WITH THE SHOCK

The most powerful initial reaction to the knowledge that you have HIV or AIDS may well be shock. If so, you could find you are in a state of extreme confusion, unable to take in information or concentrate on anything for any length of time. In that situation you may not feel up to planning ahead, gathering information or making a list of priorities for managing your life.

Shock manifests itself in a range of ways. You may be constantly in tears, or else feel very quiet and not much like talking to anyone.

You might also feel violently angry and aggressive, or very frightened and shaky. You may react calmly to the news at first, but feel very upset, scared or angry a few days later, wondering 'Why me?' and 'How did it happen?' You may simply find the news impossible to accept, or you may feel despair, or guilt, worrying about having possibly passed HIV on to other people.

It is quite possible that your life may be completely disrupted for a while. Acute insomnia or the urge to sleep the whole time, a wish to have other people constantly around or a wish to be left entirely alone are all common reactions to learning that you have HIV or AIDS. You might also feel a desire to drink, smoke and take drugs far more than usual.

On the other hand, if you have been worrying about whether you were HIV positive or likely to become ill with HIV disease, you may find that an HIV or AIDS diagnosis comes as a relief, because at least the uncertainty is over.

It is important not to ignore or neglect your feelings, even if they seem frightening and difficult to deal with. Try not to worry about what other people may think of you or how they would like you to feel; the best move you can make is to allow yourself to respond in whatever way you need. You might feel that you are coping well, that everything is under control, but then again you might feel that you should be coping 'better'. There are no 'shoulds' in such situations. If the feelings are there, they are important. Ignoring them is not going to make them go away.

Most important, you do not have to get through your initial response to a positive test result or AIDS diagnosis on your own. There are a range of ways you can get support from other people. You may be able to discuss your news with a lover, friends or family; there are also organisations which can offer counselling, advice and support (see the Directory at the back of this book for details). It might be a good idea to talk to other people with HIV or AIDS about their experiences and how they handled them. Friends with HIV could help you here, or you can meet other people with HIV and AIDS through getting in touch with a local support group. Don't worry if it seems to take a long time before you feel calm enough to make decisions or plan ahead. As far as possible, just take things one day at a time.

Getting through the first few days after an HIV or AIDS diagnosis will be a lot easier if you are getting the right medical care and attention. The next chapter looks at caring for someone with HIV illness, and *Making a Complaint*, below, discusses how to make changes if you feel you are not getting the kind of care you require. As time goes on, you may find you develop a sense that not every day will be the same. Some will be tough, others easier, and the confusion and anxiety you might be feeling at the moment will not always be with you. In time, it is likely to get a lot easier to concentrate on looking after and enjoying yourself again.

UNCERTAINTY AND INFORMATION

Everyone has to deal with a degree of uncertainty in their lives, whether or not they are living with HIV infection. Although people with AIDS are now living longer than ever before and it is far from definite that everyone with HIV infection will become ill, it is impossible to be certain what the future holds for anybody who is coping with HIV or AIDS.

It may well be pointless to try to get rid of feelings of uncertainty altogether, but it is possible to find ways to put them to one side so that they do not cast a constant shadow over your life. A good starting point might be to consider what it is you are unsure about and to think about strategies for handling the insecurity. Keeping a diary, or just writing your anxieties down as and when they occur, can help. By recording the good days as well as the bad, you can keep your feelings in some sort of perspective. Again, talking to other people with HIV and AIDS could be helpful; local support organisations are good places to take your feelings and share them, with people who are in a similar position. They are also good places to make new friends.

One of the most productive ways to deal with feelings of uncertainty is to make use of the massive amount of useful information about living with HIV that *is* available to you. Information is one of the most powerful tools you can have; do not be afraid to ask for and make use of it. If being HIV positive or having AIDS has come as a tremendous shock, it is possible that the information given to you by medical staff when you first found out made little impact. Shock and distress make it extremely hard to concentrate.

Although it is true that health staff often work under considerable pressure and do not have much time to deal with patients' concerns, you have a right to clear, accurate information about your diagnosis or antibody test result and what it may mean for you. If you cannot understand what you are being told by a doctor or nurse, say so. Ask questions if you are confused about anything. In fact, if you

151

have an appointment with your GP or a hospital doctor, it may help to write down questions that worry you in advance so that you don't forget to ask them.

Health staff are, of course, not the only source of information on HIV. Useful organisations giving information and advice on all aspects of HIV are listed in the Directory at the back of this book, some of which can also put you in contact with local agencies offering support and help. There is also a list of publications providing informative further reading.

An enormous amount can be achieved with energy, courage and the determination to stay healthy. There is no doubt that people can take steps to keep well, to set goals and meet them. Some people refer to the ideas of using positive thinking and self-help in order to stay healthy as 'self-empowerment'. There are many techniques for 'empowering' ourselves to stay well, some of which are discussed in this chapter; and in recent years considerable advances have been made in living well with HIV infection.

However, self-empowerment sometimes needs to be put in perspective. Inevitably, despite your determination to stay well, there may be times when you are ill. This can be demoralising and can drain your energy and willpower. Worrying that you are ill because you have not been determined enough to stay well can only add to your unhappiness and make it harder for you to recover. Some people call this the 'tyranny of positive thinking' - it can be a very powerful force.

If you do become ill, try to concentrate on getting through the illness as comfortably as you can. Feeling guilty is the last thing you need. Try to avoid the trap of blaming yourself and feeling that you have 'failed' in some way. You have *not* failed. Illness is sometimes unavoidable, despite our best efforts. It can be caused by more complex factors than the willpower to control your health - and your body needs rest and care so that you can start to get well again.

WHOM DO I TELL, AND HOW?

In the first few weeks after you have been given a positive test result or AIDS diagnosis, you may experience an overwhelming urge to tell everybody you know, so that you can share the feelings you have and get support. Unfortunately, the prejudice and ignorance of others can make sharing the news of your diagnosis a risky business.

Perhaps the safest rule for the time being is not to tell anyone until you are able to think clearly about who really *needs* to know and what his or her response is likely to be. If you can do this, it may well become apparent that very few people need to have information about your diagnosis or positive test result.

Sexual Partners

Being HIV positive or having AIDS does not mean you have to say no to sex. You may, however, find that your desire to have sex disappears for a while if you have recently been diagnosed HIV positive or with AIDS. This can be to do with worrying about infecting your partner(s) or a fear that you may be rejected; it can also be related to worrying about your own future. However, for many people with HIV, any loss of libido is temporary.

Speaking to sexual partners about your HIV antibody status can raise emotive issues. Deciding what to say about being HIV positive to a sexual partner involves asking yourself some tough questions. The first might be 'Does he or she *need* to know?' If you are having safer sex, you might decide you don't need to tell your partner about being HIV positive, because you are already taking steps to reduce infection risks to him or her. If you are not having safer sex, then you may want to think about ways of introducing it into your sexual relationships. You may not need to state that you are HIV positive; you could say something more general like 'I'm concerned about the kinds of infections around these days; can we agree to stick to safer sex?' Chapter 5 can provide you with some more information about making sexual relationships safer. You might also want to consider whether your partner would keep the information confidential.

There are of course other reasons for wanting to tell partners about your being HIV positive or having an AIDS diagnosis. You may be in a long-term relationship where your partner already knows that you have HIV, and who will thus be able to offer you support, encouragement and practical help if he or she knows about your diagnosis. You may be at the start of a relationship which looks as though it could be important to you, and feel that you want to be clear with your partner from the beginning about your antibody status. Or you may feel that you would rather tell your partner at an early stage of your HIV infection so that you can be clear about whether or not you can expect support from him or her later on.

Not telling your partner about being HIV positive may have serious implications in some situations; for example, if you are planning to have a baby together. In such a situation, having unsafe sex in order for pregnancy to occur could put your partner at risk, and there is also a risk of the baby becoming infected with HIV before birth. If you are in a stable relationship, and think it likely that you have become HIV positive through sex or unsafe drug use with another person (of whom your partner is not aware), your position will be more difficult.

There are no easy answers to such problems. You may find it helpful to talk them through with a counsellor (see Chapter 8) or a support group. Contacting a local or national HIV helpline may also be useful. Getting as much information as you can to deal with your own and your partner's questions about HIV (if you do decide to tell him or her) will help. This will take time; but you need time to consider the important issues involved. Thinking in advance about ways of handling your partner's possible reactions may be helpful. However, it is possible that the situation cannot be resolved without some degree of pain and distress to you or your partner. You may have to come to terms with this.

Family and Friends

Sometimes, family and friends are the first source of support people turn to in difficult times. On the other hand, you may not have a particularly close relationship with your family. If you are gay or bisexual and have not told your family or friends, you may be afraid to tell them you are HIV positive because they might ask about your sexuality at the same time. Of course, you do not have to tell any friends or family members if you do not want to. However, there is no doubt that if you decide to do so, getting advice and information about this first can make an enormous difference to the way your news is received.

Health Care Staff

You may feel that your dentist, surgeon or GP should know that you have HIV because they will need to protect themselves from infection. In fact, health staff should be routinely taking steps to stay safe from infection anyway. On the other hand, not telling your GP about being HIV positive may make it difficult for you to get the early care and treatment that can help to keep you healthy. If you have been diagnosed with HIV-related illness by a hospital doctor, it might be important for your GP to know so that he or she can give you appropriate medical attention. However, no one has the right to inform your GP unless you give specific consent for this to happen.

It is important that you are happy that health staff with whom you deal are properly informed of the need for confidentiality. If you have concerns about how information about your test result or diagnosis will be handled, you could speak to your hospital or clinic doctor about this. Ask what the options are, and let him or her know clearly whom you want and do not want told. The doctor should make sure that, when hospital care is necessary, it will be provided by staff who are well-informed, discreet and supportive. If you are worried that your GP will pass information about your seropositivity to other people (such as family members, for example), ask for help with finding another GP on whom you can rely to maintain confidentiality.

At Work

Deciding whether to tell people at work about your diagnosis or positive test result raises another set of issues. There is no risk of HIV infection in the workplace through sitting or speaking to others, sharing toilet facilities, coffee cups, cigarettes and so on. Unless you are practising unsafe sex or drug use with colleagues, or health and safety measures for dealing with spilled blood are inadequate (see Chapter 4), your HIV-positive status does not represent a risk to other people at work.

Even with accurate information and training about HIV infection, some colleagues may still feel threatened by and hostile towards people with HIV. HIV-positive people have been sacked, suspended or pressured into leaving because colleagues were afraid of becoming infected.

At work, as elsewhere, the 'need to know' principle applies. If you feel that there are specific people at work who are well-informed enough about HIV to offer you confidential support, that may be helpful. Not all companies behave badly towards people with HIV or AIDS. Some have shown sensitivity, kindness and concern towards HIV-positive people employed by them, making generous sick leave and financial support available where necessary. You may be lucky enough to work for a company like this. If you are unsure, it will probably help to seek advice on the matter; organisations listed in the Directory at the back of this book can help you. *Dealing with Employment Difficulties Related to HIV* later in this chapter gives further information.

KEEPING AN EYE ON YOUR HEALTH

As most illnesses are more effectively dealt with if treated at an early stage, it may help for you to monitor your health so that you are aware of any changes as early as possible and can get appropriate medical help. Early treatment of related infections and watching out for signs of a damaged immune system are both excellent ways of preventing HIV disease.

Keeping an eye on your health may involve a range of measures, some of which you can do on your own while others require the help and guidance of your GP or hospital doctor; these are discussed below. Another benefit of taking steps to monitor your health is that it can have a strong psychological benefit: you will be attuned to the 'ups' and 'downs' your body may go through and will know that periods of ill-health do not mean that you will never feel healthy again. In other words, you will be playing an active and powerful role in living well with HIV infection.

Staying in touch with changes in the health of your body is not, however, the same thing as constantly checking and re-checking for symptoms of illness. If you think that monitoring your health is likely to become an obsessive process of hunting for evidence that you are ill, try talking to a counsellor or to friends, or learning techniques for relaxation (see *Managing Stress*, below).

Drug Use and HIV Infection

Drug use, like HIV infection, is an emotive issue where stereotypes prevail. Prejudice against people with HIV who use drugs may, therefore, be particularly strong. If you find you have to cope with the misinformed assumptions of others about people who use drugs it may well be tiring, stressful and alienating, none of which is likely to help you to live well with HIV infection.

There may also be other problems to deal with. You might find it more difficult to practise safer sex when you are taking drugs. Having unsafe sex can put you at risk not only of sexual infections such as gonorrhoea or chlamydia but of other strains of HIV infection, all of which may weaken your immune system further. Chapter 5 can give you more information about staying safe in sexual relationships and protecting your partners.

Using street drugs can suppress your immune system because of their impurity, and drugs such as alcohol and nicotine also act as immuno-suppressants, making it harder to stay well with HIV infection. In addition, there are risks of septicaemia and hepatitis B from sharing works. Chapter 4 gives you detailed information about safer drug use.

If you feel that drug use is the most significant part of your life, other things, like having a comfortable and safe place to live, eating and sleeping well, can start to seem far less important. You might not have the time or the energy to think about them. However, being able to rest, relax and eat well are very important aspects of staying healthy with HIV infection.

Remember that you do not have to cope with these kinds of worries on your own. You may feel that you have enough information and support to live well with HIV as a drug user. If you do not, the range of services available to people who use drugs are described in Chapter 4. Some of these may also be able to provide you with advice and help on HIV matters; other agencies dealing with drug and HIV issues are detailed in the Directory at the back of this book.

Keeping a Diary

Recording the way you feel physically and mentally on a regular basis might be a useful measure. A diary of this kind can help you recall early symptoms of illnesses you may have already experienced, so that you will recognise them should they recur. It may also help you to remember basic measures you might have taken previously to deal with ill health, which could serve you well again.

Getting Information

Care and treatment for people with HIV-related illness may involve a combination of blood and organ tests (see below) and drugs to deal with both the infections related to HIV and the action of the virus on your body. Your GP, hospital or clinic doctor will be responsible for providing this care and treatment, and in theory this should be based on the best expertise and information available. However, standards of care for people with HIV illness vary considerably, and you may wish to reassure yourself about the relevance of any tests being conducted and treatments administered. Taking an active role in your care by getting as much information as you can could also boost your morale and help you to take appropriate steps to get over illness as quickly as possible.

Knowing the right questions to ask your doctor is the first stage in this process. There are now a range of excellent newsletters available on treatment issues, written by and for people with HIV, many of which are cheap or free. Further details about relevant publications and organisations to contact are listed in the Directory at the back of this book.

Check-ups and Tests

Medical check-ups are a good way of keeping in touch with your state of health. People with HIV but no symptoms of illness might consider having a check-up every three to six months, people with HIV illness around once a month to every six weeks. A thorough check-up involves not only a proper examination of your mouth, abdomen, chest and nervous system but also an update on any recent changes in your health. Feel free to volunteer information that may be useful; this is particularly important if you are experiencing symptoms such as breathlessness, chest pains, bowel or mouth discomfort, and so on.

Generally, a medical check-up for a person with HIV will also include tests to see whether your body's immune system has been damaged by the virus. These might include *HIV antibody and antigen tests*. A *biochemical profile* checks your blood to see whether metabolic processes are working properly, and a *full blood count* involves a computerised count of the red and white blood cells and platelets in your blood. These can change not only as a result of HIV infection but also through other infections, nutritional deficiencies, and so on.

If you are a woman with HIV, it is helpful to have regular cervical smears. You can also check your breasts regularly, by feeling them carefully with the flat of your hand once a month (it helps if you raise the left arm when you feel the left breast, and vice versa). If you do this regularly, you will soon get used to the way your breasts feel, and will notice if there are any unusual lumps. This is good advice for all women, not just women with HIV.

There are a number of other tests used to monitor your immune system or check for particular HIV-related infections. There is no space to describe these in detail here, but it is important to ask your doctor what they involve. Some may cause you discomfort (such as invasive techniques like a *bronchoscopy*, for which an instrument used to examine your lungs enters via your nose), and you may want to be prepared for this. You may want to be provided with enough information so that you can decide whether the benefits such techniques might provide are worth the discomfort.

Eating Well

A healthy diet means different things to different people. Some people with HIV may take a very active interest in nutrition and stick very carefully to a particular diet, while others may live mainly off convenience foods and take-aways. As far as HIV infection is concerned, there is no proof that any one approach to eating will keep you healthy. What you eat is, in any case, dictated by how much money you have to buy food, how much time you can spend preparing it, and whether or not you have the willpower and inclination to follow a strictly controlled regime.

As with other approaches to self-help, what is good for you is largely a question of what is realistic and what you feel comfortable with. If struggling to eat only those foods you identify as healthy is going to cause you stress and give rise to cravings for chocolate, cakes and chips, then indulging yourself from time to time is probably going to do you more good than trying to ignore your cravings.

On the other hand, a diet of junk food is unlikely to benefit your health in the long term. Most vitamins and minerals you need are available from a mixture of fresh foods, including a good range of fruits, vegetables, nuts, grains and pulses. Some of the publications listed in the Directory at the back of this book can give you further information on healthy eating, or you could ask your GP or doctor at your local clinic to give you details of a dietitian. There may be a special reason why a doctor would prescribe extra vitamins or minerals, but generally there is no proof that these are useful if you are eating a well-balanced diet.

Food-poisoning is always unpleasant, but for a person with weakened immunity it can be very serious. You can take steps to avoid it by making sure that fruit and vegetables are cleaned before you eat them, and that meats, fish, poultry or re-heated foods are cooked properly all the way through. If you go abroad it may be best to avoid fresh salads and fruit in countries where the water is not clean enough to drink, and to stick to foods that have been cooked thoroughly.

Sleeping Well

Everybody needs a different amount of sleep to function properly, and most of us can make do with less sleep for short periods if we are able to recuperate the lost hours from time to time. While there is no set number of hours required by a person with HIV to stay healthy, it is important to respect your body's need for sleep and try to balance day- and night-time activities so that you can enjoy yourself and fulfil social and work commitments without getting run-down and exhausted. Lack of sleep stresses your immune system as well as diminishing your energy. It may also have a psychological effect: problems and anxieties can seem harder to manage when we are tired.

Unfortunately, becoming fixated with getting the right amount of sleep can sometimes have the effect of causing stress and keeping you awake. Try not to worry if this happens. There are a number of ways to cope with insomnia, ranging from a cup of cocoa and a good book to practising relaxation techniques (see *Learning to Relax*, below). Sleeping pills may help temporarily, but they are not a long-term solution and may be harmful if you find you cannot manage without them. Sleeping well at night may also be easier if you can take exercise fairly regularly each day. How feasible this is will depend on your state of health, but staying as fit as you can may help you to 'switch off' properly when you go to bed.

Taking Exercise

Regular exercise will help you to stay healthy, and may help you to feel good. As well as improving your strength and stamina, exercise feeds internal organs through improved circulation, and may have a beneficial effect on the immune system. A person who works his or her body through an appropriate exercise programme is often able to relax better, and may also look better, than someone who never takes exercise. Feeling good about your body and following a manageable routine may also boost your self-confidence and willpower.

What and how much you do is up to you. If you are unused to taking a lot of exercise, start gently. The most important thing is to set yourself realistic targets, and to do things you enjoy. There is nothing so off-putting as aiming so high that you constantly fall short of your own expectations, or participating in a sport which you don't particularly like but feel is 'good for you'.

You may be able to build exercise into your daily routine: walking, jogging or cycling to work or to a friend's house when you normally take the bus, for example. If you cannot get out much, there are very simple exercises you can do. Try individually tensing the different muscles in your legs, arms, buttocks, shoulders, feet, hands and face, then slowly relaxing them. You might also like to try rotating your hands, feet, legs, arms, and head.

Taking Care at Home

Staying healthy with HIV does not mean that you will need to take a vast number of special hygienic precautions at home. What you do may be the same as what anybody, HIV negative or positive, would do to avoid infections. The following suggestions are a few common-sense measures for good domestic and personal care.

- Dirty clothes, linen and so on can be washed in the hot cycle of a washing machine. There is no need to keep these separate from other people's laundry. If clothing, towels or bed linen has been heavily stained with body fluids, you may also want to soak them in bleach or boil them for a short while. Make sure you follow any washing instructions on the label of the item.
- Keep different cleaning cloths for use in the kitchen and bathroom. If body fluids such as blood are spilled, mop them up with tissues and throw the tissues away (if the fluids are from someone else's body, wear household gloves to clean up the spillage). A bleach solution of one part bleach to ten parts water is adequate to inactivate HIV in spillages.
- Try to keep your fridge, bread-bin and other food containers clean and mould-free by regularly cleaning them with hot water. If you have kept food in the fridge for more than three days, it might be best to throw it away. Frozen food should be defrosted properly, and reheated food cooked thoroughly.
- Make sure you wash your hands after using the toilet. It also helps to wash your hands before preparing and eating food.
- If you can, have a bath or shower daily. Apart from the obvious benefits of feeling refreshed and clean, this can avoid infections. Avoid sharing toothbrushes and razors.
- Used tampons and tissues can be disposed of safely down the toilet. Sanitary towels and medical dressings can be wrapped in a plastic bag and thrown away (tie up the opening of the bag first). Used condoms can be wrapped in a bag or bit of paper and thrown away (flushing them down the toilet can sometimes block drains).
- Keep your teeth and gums as clean as possible. A hard toothbrush can hurt your gums, so a soft one may be better. Dental floss or toothpicks can help keep gums clean and prevent tooth decay – but use them carefully as they can cut sensitive gums. If you have mouth ulcers or sores of any sort, you may prefer to use cotton wool buds to clean your teeth and gums until they clear up.

- If you cut or graze yourself, clean the wound immediately under running water and try to allow it to bleed a little (this helps rinse out germs). Antiseptic and a waterproof plaster should prevent further infection. For more serious injuries, always get medical help.

Domestic Animals

Your pet should be checked by the vet for any communicable diseases (*toxoplasmosis gondii*, for example, can be in dirty cat litter - see Chapter 2), and always wear rubber gloves when cleaning up faeces or urine. Rubber gloves should also be worn for cleaning bird cages, aquariums and cat litters, which can be disinfected regularly with a solution of one part bleach to ten parts water. If you've been touching your pet take care always to wash your hands before you handle food. It is probably not a good idea to let your pet lick your face, as germs can be transmitted from its mouth to yours. Feeding your animal cooked meat will prevent the possibility of transmission of the parasites that live in raw flesh.

Managing Stress

Feelings that build up over a period of time without being expressed may end up causing severe stress. This section looks at ways of 'letting go' of feelings and unwinding so that your body can rest and relax.

Stress is not necessarily destructive. Sometimes we are able to channel feelings of being pressurised and unrelaxed into something creative, such as hard physical exercise, the completion of a difficult piece of work, and so on. However, if it is more likely that stress will simply accumulate and drain your energy rather than increase it, the following suggestions may be useful.

- Keep communicating: The idea that you have to hide your feelings will not only stop you from being able to work through them, it will also mean that other people will assume you are all right when you are not. Bottling up feelings is exhausting and can be terribly lonely. On the other hand, talking to friends or a counsellor may seem frightening, but it is almost never as difficult as you might think it will be.
- Write down what makes you feel bad: If you can identify the situations that cause you misery or anger, try writing them down. This can have a number of effects: you will have a concrete idea

of what is bothering you, which can be far more helpful than worries churning endlessly in your head. Sometimes just the act of writing down what worries you can make it more manageable. The next stage is deciding which stresses are inevitable (in which case the relaxation techniques mentioned below may help) and which you can take action to reduce or avoid.

- Silence your private judge: Many of us carry around what could be called a 'private judge' in our heads, that voice which comments on our behaviour in a critical and negative manner. People with a forceful private judge may have low self-esteem, so that they can only see their mistakes and are unable to accept praise for their achievements. The judging voice that tells you that HIV infection is your fault, that 'not coping' with HIV illness means you are a failure, and deserve to be ill, is one that needs to be silenced.

  Some people have found it helpful to counter automatic negative thoughts such as 'It's my fault I'm ill; I didn't eat well/sleep well/exercise well enough', or 'I don't see X as much as before; s/he is probably avoiding me because I have HIV' by focussing on a positive statement instead. For example: 'Being ill is tough, but I know I can get through this situation', or 'X might be finding it difficult to make time to see me at the moment; I'll give him/her a ring and see if we can work something out.'

  It is important to emphasise here that considering a positive as well as a negative interpretation of any situation concerns breaking out of automatic self-critical patterns of thought. It does not mean sitting on hurt feelings or anger in the hopes that they will go away if you ignore them or because you are afraid that they are foolish or invalid in some way. If a situation or person has upset you, then that feeling is real and not foolish. Discussing it with someone you know and trust may well be a good idea (see 'Keep Communicating', above).

- Avoid 'musturbating': This is quite different from masturbating, which can be an excellent way to relieve stress. *Musturbating* is what we do when we set ourselves impossible goals, or see our lives in prohibitively black-and-white terms. It is a process which has been described as making agreements with ourselves along the following lines: 'I *must* remember to always be optimistic about being HIV positive, or I'll upset other people', or 'I *must* make a point of always asking other people their news first, or they'll think I'm obsessed with having AIDS'. Similar to musturbating is 'awfulising'; for example: 'It would be *awful* if I

163

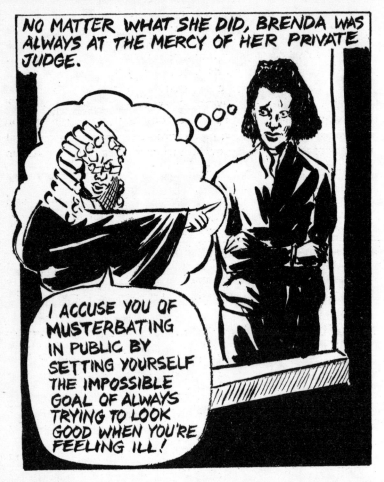

allowed people to know how ill I feel', or 'It would be *awful* if my lover found out how afraid I am of losing him/her because of my HIV infection'.

Living with HIV is difficult enough without such unrealistic and pointless self-imposed pressures. If you are a musturbator or an awfuliser, you are not alone: almost everyone puts pressure on him- or herself in this way to a greater or lesser degree. Joining a local support group might enable you to find out how other people with HIV have found ways of avoiding stress of this sort. Talking to a counsellor, friend, or your lover might also be a helpful way of distinguishing the worthwhile and important goals from those that are not.

Learning to Relax

There are a great variety of techniques for letting go of tension and allowing your body to sink into a rested, peaceful state. If you are unused to making time to relax, it is a skill that may take a little time to acquire. Focussing on restful thoughts or images and excluding stressful ones may not always be easy at first, but it will become more effective with practice. Some approaches to relaxation are looked at briefly below; publications listed in the Directory at the back of this book will provide much more thorough information on the subject.

- Do something you enjoy: Reading a book, lying down and listening to a favourite piece of music, going for a walk or out to a film or play may all be relaxing activities if they make you happy and help you to switch off for a while. Similarly, developing the skill of saying 'no' without guilt to activities and occasions which do not interest you (but which you were considering in order to make another person happy) can be wonderfully relaxing.
- Tensing and stretching: Begin by sitting in a comfortable chair or lying down in a quiet room; make sure your entire body is supported. Close your eyes and concentrate on your breathing so that you become aware of its rhythm. Just listen to your breathing for a few minutes. The next stage is to focus on all the different muscles in your body, from your feet right up to your face. Slowly tense each set of muscles in turn, then relax them. As you tense, breathe in and hold the tension for two counts. Then, as you breathe out again, relax the muscles. Let the tension rush out, and keep breathing naturally. It may help to say the word 'relax' to yourself quietly as you breathe out.

  Remember to tense only one group of muscles at a time, and do not strain to make them as tight as they will go (this might lead to cramp). Tighten them only as much as you feel comfortable with: this will get easier with practice.
- Visualisation: This technique can work well if preceded by the above tensing and stretching exercise. Sit or lie in a quiet, darkened room and breathe deeply in and out of your nose for a few minutes. Concentrate on your breathing. If other thoughts come into your head, do not struggle to ignore them, but do not allow them to distract you. Let them come and go. After three or four minutes, focus on a memory or image that relaxes you

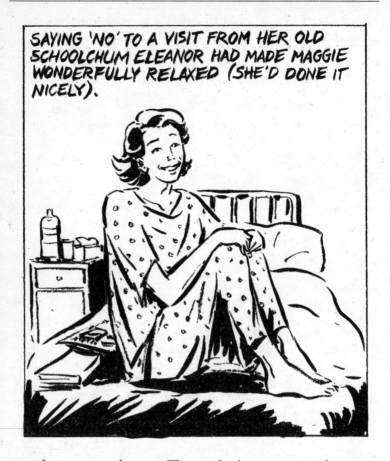

SAYING 'NO' TO A VISIT FROM HER OLD SCHOOLCHUM ELEANOR HAD MADE MAGGIE WONDERFULLY RELAXED (SHE'D DONE IT NICELY).

and gives you pleasure. This might be an image of a warm summer's day – you are lying on a sandy beach or in some long grass in a field full of beautiful flowers. Try to imagine the sights, sounds and impressions around you: a bird-song, the warmth of the sun on your face and body, the colours, shapes and smells of the flowers. Allow yourself to soak all this up, feeling all the tension and tightness leave your body. See if you can float into this image, and experience it fully.

Five to ten minutes will be long enough for this exercise at first. When you have finished, lie still for a few minutes and let yourself gradually become aware of your surroundings again. When you are ready, get up slowly and smoothly.

• Massage: There is little space in a book of this sort to give details of massage as a relaxation technique. Many people find receiving a massage to be a wonderful release of tension; learning to massage your own face, shoulders, neck and other parts of your body can also be very soothing. A local or national HIV agency may be able to provide details of people who provide massage (sometimes specifically for people with HIV and AIDS) in your area.

ALTERNATIVE MEDICINE

In Chapter 2, details of the different drugs available for treating HIV-related illness and dealing with the direct impact of the virus upon the immune system were discussed.

Conventional medicine on its own, however, may be unable to provide a universally effective treatment for a life-threatening infection such as HIV. The improvements that drug therapies may bring about are often countered by unpleasant side-effects, and even if clinical drugs are successful in treating a particular infection, they cannot take into account the health of the whole body (i.e. take a 'holistic' approach).

Views about the validity of alternative or complementary therapies are deeply divided. Some people believe that conventional medicine is ineffective because it tends to deal with symptoms alone, whereas alternative therapies aim to include the social and personal circumstances that can cause illness (of course, every good doctor should take into account the effects of stress caused to a patient by, say, relationship difficulties, or an inability to confront and deal with feelings). Other people think of alternative therapies as an expensive waste of time, strictly for cranks and hypochondriacs.

Finally, there is a growing body of people who do not regard conventional and alternative therapies as mutually exclusive. For them, it is a question of exploring ways of balancing and benefiting from both. The fact that medical practitioners increasingly feature in this group suggests that providers of conventional medicine are beginning to broaden their outlook on health care.

The arrival of HIV is likely to have played a significant role in any increase in the credibility of alternative therapies. Since there is no conventional drug that can be said to cure HIV infection, people who are HIV positive may wish to be given as much information as possible about other treatment options. They may wish to question what they are told by medical practitioners; they may wish to take more responsibility for their own health care.

Whether or not you feel that alternatives to conventional

medicine may offer you any health benefits is a personal matter, and needs very careful consideration. Brief information is given here on some of the available therapies, and further relevant publications and helpful organisations are listed in the Directory at the back of this book. If you are considering following a particular therapy, it may well be helpful to try and get further advice from someone who has tried it (a friend with HIV or a member of your support group, for example).

It is also important to talk to your doctor, since the treatment may be available on the NHS, and because some alternative therapies do not interact well with conventional treatments. Even if your doctor does not agree with the idea of alternative therapies, he or she is obliged to provide you with relevant information. Similarly, if you are considering trying more than one alternative treatment, it's a good idea to discuss this with the therapist, as some therapies can block each other from working (such as acupuncture and homoeopathy, for example). Some of the possible pros and cons of taking alternative treatments are discussed briefly below.

Some Possible Advantages of Trying Alternative Therapies
- Many people with HIV use alternative therapies. The most obvious advantage is that these may be effective in halting the action of HIV upon the body, or in preventing related infections.
- Even if there is no conclusive evidence that some therapies are effective, individuals who use them may feel and look better because they *believe* them to be effective. This may sound like a fraudulent argument; however there is little doubt that for many people, believing that a treatment is going to improve their health is the first stage in the process of recovery (this applies equally to the success of conventional methods).
- Exploring a range of treatment options and gathering as much information about these as possible can help people with HIV feel they are taking control of their situation and adopting a positive approach to living with the virus. Such an approach may very well have beneficial effects upon an individual's health.

Some Possible Disadvantages of Trying Alternative Therapies
- As stated above, some therapies may interact badly with conventional treatments. Other therapies may get in the way of your diet, so that you may need to change your eating patterns or what you eat.
- Many alternative therapies remain untested. In 1990,

investigative journalist Duncan Campbell exposed a number of practitioners selling untested 'treatments' for people with HIV in the UK. Some of these proved to be ineffective but harmless; others were found to be downright dangerous. While only a small minority of practitioners of alternative treatments are likely to be dishonest or incompetent, it is always worth getting further advice about a treatment (if possible from someone who has already tried it) if you feel in the least unsure about it.

• Some therapists charge enormous amounts for their services. That may rule them out entirely from the point of view of a person on a low income. However, it may be a good idea to check and compare prices, as there is sometimes an extraordinary disparity in fees charged by different therapists offering the same or similar treatment. Some therapists operate on a 'sliding scale' basis so that people with a higher income pay more than those with a lower or no income at all. Whatever the charge for a particular treatment, the most important point is that the person receiving it should feel that it is worth it.

Some Alternative Therapies

The following information is in no sense a comprehensive guide to all the therapies available, neither does it necessarily imply a recommendation of those mentioned. In reaching a decision about whether to try an alternative treatment, you will need to seek further information and guidance, for instance from the publications and organisations listed in the Directory at the back of this book.

Visualisation and *massage* are both discussed above. They can reduce stress and help people to relax, bringing about feelings of well-being and comfort.

Acupuncture

Acupuncture works on the principle that energy flows through the body in lines (called *Meridians*), which are blocked by specific illnesses. Very sharp needles are inserted into the body at particular points to unblock the energy. Acupuncture can be very relaxing, and may play a significant role in relieving symptoms of illness. If you are considering trying it, it is a good idea to buy your own needles – the clinic will be able to help you – as sharing these carries risks of HIV infection through contact with infected blood. Many clinics now use disposable needles anyway – check with the clinic.

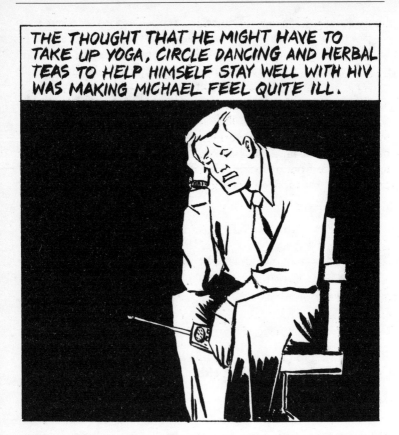

THE THOUGHT THAT HE MIGHT HAVE TO TAKE UP YOGA, CIRCLE DANCING AND HERBAL TEAS TO HELP HIMSELF STAY WELL WITH HIV WAS MAKING MICHAEL FEEL QUITE ILL.

Aromatherapy

Aromatherapy is based on the idea that smells can have a positive effect on the psyche, and thus on the body. Aromatherapists generally practise massage using a range of different scented oils, which are considered to have different properties (their primary aim being to reduce tension and stress and induce a sense of well-being).

Homoeopathy

Homoeopathy works on the principles that what causes symptoms of illness in someone healthy can cure symptoms in someone ill, and that the smallest possible dose of such a substance is all that is necessary to make the therapy effective. Although toxic substances are used, they are at such infinitesimal dosages that toxicity does not seem to occur. It is important not to try to treat yourself with homoeopathic medicines; practitioners are trained to get the dosage levels absolutely right for the particular individual being treated and his or her specific symptoms of disease.

Vitamin and Mineral Supplements
These are considered important to help the body's metabolism. There is, however, little evidence to support the idea that unlimited amounts of additional vitamins and minerals are helpful to the body: at best, any excess will be lost from the body, and at worst, toxicity may occur. On the other hand, taking measured amounts of vitamins and minerals may help some people. The best idea is to get advice from a doctor, who may also be able to give you a prescription for moderate dosages of relevant pills.

Getting Help from Community Carers

In addition to the medical care available to people with HIV and AIDS - GPs, GU clinics and hospitals as discussed in this chapter and in Chapter 6 - there are a range of services offering information, advice and practical help in your area if you need them. These are discussed more fully in Chapter 8, under *Community Health Services*.

HANDLING PRACTICAL ISSUES

Financial Support

The following section looks at the main Social Security and other benefits which people with HIV illness and the people who care for them can claim. It may also be possible to get financial assistance from a range of organisations which make grants to people with HIV-related illness and AIDS; some of these are listed in the Directory at the back of this book.

This book cannot give details of all relevant benefits, and of the eligibility criteria involved. Regulations governing benefit provision are very complex; if you think you may be eligible for any of the range of benefits mentioned, you can get further advice and guidance on the matter. Sometimes applying for a particular benefit can be a complicated job, and there are organisations to help you with making applications as well as by giving general information (see the Directory for details).

Finally, fears about lack of confidentiality have put some people off claiming benefits to which they were entitled. It may help to check with the Department of Social Security (DSS) that no one will be told of your HIV antibody status without your prior consent.

Please note that where eligibility criteria refer to partnerships this applies to heterosexual relationships only; the Department of Social Security does not include gay and lesbian couples in the definition of a sexual partnership.

All information given below is accurate at the time of writing. However, whereas broad eligibility criteria are likely to remain fixed, the amount of savings you may be allowed when claiming a means-tested benefit is likely to change from levels set in April 1991. It is therefore important to get further, up-to-date information from the relevant organisations.

People Who Are Unemployed

To qualify for *Unemployment Benefit*, a weekly sum payable for up to 12 months of unemployment, you need to have paid adequate National Insurance (NI) contributions, to be seen to be unemployed through no fault of your own, and to be available for and actively seeking work.

Living on a Low Income

If you have no income or are on a low income there are a range of benefits which you can claim. The amount available varies according to your circumstances; whether you are single or living with a heterosexual partner, for example, and the amount of income you and your partner are already receiving.

You can claim *Income Support* if:

- You are over 18 (or over 16 if you are unfit for work, or fit into another special category)
- The Social Security office assesses that you receive no income or are on a low income
- Neither you nor your partner has joint savings of more than £8000 or is working for 16 hours or more a week.

Income support is supposed to provide you with a level of income legally defined as appropriate to your circumstances.

If you are on a low income, pay rent and have savings of less than £16,000, you may be entitled to some *Housing Benefit*. How much you get may depend on your level of income and savings, and your particular circumstances. Similarly if you have to pay the Community Charge (Poll Tax), you should get help with this.

If you or your partner are receiving Attendance Allowance,

Mobility Allowance, Invalidity Benefit, or Severe Disablement Allowance (see below), or are registered as a blind person, you will automatically get a *Disability Premium* included in the assessment of your Income Support, Housing Benefit or Poll Tax Benefit. You should also get the Disability Premium if you have been registered as sick for 28 weeks. The amount varies according to whether you are single or living with someone.

If you or your partner are working 16 hours or more a week, have savings of no more than £8000, and have at least one dependent child under 16 (or between 16 and 19 in full-time education to the equivalent of A level), you will be able to claim *Family Credit*. Again, the amount you get will depend on the level of net income in your relationship, and the number and ages of your children. Payments will be made for 26 weeks, after which you will need to re-apply.

Taking Time Off Work Due to Sickness
If you are working for an employer, *Statutory Sick Pay* is paid (after tax and National Insurance have been deducted) by your employer for up to 28 weeks of leave from work due to sickness. You have to be ill for four or more days in a row to qualify. Spells of sickness which count towards the 28 weeks must be no more than eight weeks apart. *Occupational Sick Pay* is also paid by many employers, and Statutory Sick Pay will be included within it.

If you are unemployed, or self-employed with sufficient NI contributions, or employed but not eligible for Statutory Sick Pay, you may qualify for *Sickness Benefit*, a payment made for up to 28 weeks of illness. As with Statutory Sick Pay, spells of illness counting towards the 28 weeks must be no more than eight weeks apart.

If you are away from work due to sickness for over 28 weeks, and were previously either employed, self-employed, or unemployed with adequate NI contributions, you should be able to get *Invalidity Benefit*. Payment of Invalidity Benefit should be automatic for people who have received sickness benefit for 28 weeks.

If you did not pay adequate NI contributions and you have been incapable of work for at least 28 weeks, *Severe Disablement Allowance* may be available for people aged 16 or over. People of 20 years and over have, however, found it difficult to get this. For people who are unlikely to be able to return to work through disability or sickness, *Occupational Pension* is offered by a range of employers, including public service and nationalised industries, the Civil Service and some private companies. This is given in addition to State contributory benefits.

People with Haemophilia

Payments on behalf of people with haemophilia and HIV have been made by the Government into a fund administered by the MacFarlane Trust. Payments to meet special needs are available, and should not affect claims for *Income Support* or *Housing Benefit*. Details of the MacFarlane Trust are given in the Directory at the back of this book.

Pregnant Women and Mothers with HIV

If you have worked full-time with your employer for 2 years up to 15 weeks before your baby is expected, *Statutory Maternity Pay* is paid for 18 weeks after you have left work. To qualify for it, you need to stop working at any point between 11 and 6 weeks before your baby is due. If you have not worked long enough with the employer but have paid adequate National Insurance contributions, you may be eligible for *Maternity Allowance*, which is payable for 18 weeks after you stop work (again, this has to be between 11 and 6 weeks before your baby is due). If you receive *Income Support* or *Family Credit* (see above), you will be eligible for a lump sum called *Maternity Payment*. This comes from the *Social Fund* (see below).

During the time of pregnancy and for 12 months after the birth you will also qualify for free prescriptions and dental treatment.

Everyone with a child under 16 (or under 19 if in full-time education) is entitled to *Child Benefit*. If you are a single parent, you may be eligible for *One Parent Benefit*, a payment for the eldest child only, on top of Child Benefit. An unmarried parent (even if living with a partner) who is looking after a child can get the additional Personal Tax Allowance.

Needing Someone to Look after You

You may be able to get the new *Disability Living Allowance* if you have difficulty walking and/or if you need some looking after at home from another person. The Disability Living Allowance replaced *Attendance Allowance* and *Mobility Allowance* in April 1992. There are special rules for people who are terminally ill. For more details contact a Welfare Rights Advisor.

Blindness or Partial Sight

Registering with your local Social Services Department as a blind or partially-sighted person means that you may get a range of benefits, including Severe Disablement Allowance and Income Support. Proof from an eye specialist will, however, be necessary.

Being Cared for Outside Home or Hospital
If you go into a nursing home, hospice or residential care and have savings of less than £8000, Income Support will boost your income to help towards covering residential care or a nursing home (it must be one registered with the local Council).

Grants and Loans
The Social Fund provides grants and interest-free loans to people on Income Support to help them meet the cost of items like furniture, clothing and funeral expenses. Whether or not you will get a grant or loan depends very much on the set of priorities in your local DSS office, and how healthy its budget is. It makes sense to get advice before applying.

Looking after Someone Else
If you are under pensionable age, spend at least 35 hours a week caring for someone who is getting Attendance Allowance, and do not earn more than £40, you may well qualify for *Invalid Care Allowance*. (However, this is not payable if you are getting an equivalent or higher amount of money already from other benefits.) You may also qualify for Income Support.

Following a Death
Money is available from the Social Fund to cover the cost of a funeral. It is payable to anyone who has to arrange a funeral and is getting any one of a range of benefits, including Income Support, Family Credit or Housing Benefit.

If You Are Widowed
A range of benefits are available to women who are widowed; a few are also available to widowers. There is an income tax allowance called *Widow's Bereavement Allowance* for the tax year of the husband's death and the year following. If there is a dependent child, a widow or widower can get an additional tax allowance, and there is also a *Widowed Mother's Allowance* payable to widows with dependent children. *Widow's Pensions* are available to people aged 45 or over without dependent children.

A lump sum payment called *Widow's Payment* can be claimed by widows under 60, or aged 60 if their late husband was not receiving a retirement pension. It may also be possible to get an additional pension on your late husband's earnings since 1978, if he was making contributions to the State Earnings-related Pension

Scheme. Occupational pension schemes often pay a pension to a widow, and sometimes to widowers.

Housing

Being homeless or having inadequate housing can cause all kinds of problems for people with HIV. Not having a secure place to live can cause severe stress, and if housing is inappropriate (for example, if it is cold, or damp, or has inadequate washing or cooking facilities) it can trigger or exacerbate illness. Everyone is entitled to accommodation which is warm, secure, private, comfortable and affordable. If you have HIV and are having difficulties finding or keeping such accommodation, this section may offer some useful basic information. However, it cannot deal with all your concerns, so you will need to contact the housing agencies listed in the Directory at the back of this book for further help.

A national shortage of housing generally does not help the situation for people who may have special needs related to health problems. The prejudice and ignorance of owners, caretakers or neighbours has meant that some people with HIV have been evicted from rented accommodation. Finally, it is very difficult for voluntary or statutory agencies to provide help and support for people with HIV or AIDS who do not have somewhere secure to live, because they have no fixed address.

Finding a Place to Live

If you are homeless, or will soon become homeless, you should contact your local Council. Housing policy varies enormously from one region to another, so it is a good idea to get advice from a law centre, advice bureau or relevant voluntary organisation.

The 1985 Housing Act Part III imposes statutory obligations on local authorities to assist homeless people on condition they fulfil certain criteria, such as 'priority need'. The law states that people in priority need include pregnant women or women with dependent children. Others might be in priority need because they are 'vulnerable' in some way, for example through old age, mental illness, physical handicap or disability, or, as the law puts it, for 'some other special reason'.

Unfortunately, in some boroughs, people with HIV who have no symptoms of illness may not be considered in 'priority need' and will have a hard time obtaining accommodation from the local

Council. There is also no obligation for a local authority to re-house permanently a person who is considered to have made him- or herself 'intentionally' homeless, although temporary accommodation should be made available. If you have applied to the local authority for accommodation, and are considered to be either not homeless, or intentionally homeless, it is important to get independent advice immediately (see the Directory). It is also the case that if you have no local connection in the area of the Council you have approached they do not have to rehouse you permanently themselves. It is their duty, however, to provide you with temporary accommodation and then refer you to the area where you have the strongest local connection, unless you have no local connection elsewhere.

When you apply to the Council for housing, your application will generally be dealt with by the Homeless Person's Unit, or by the Emergency Housing Office. Medical records from a hospital or GP may be required if you are applying as a 'vulnerable' person, as will details of where you have lived for the past five years. If you are worried that information about your health will be shared without your consent, you could insist that it be confined only to workers within the authority who need to know in order to assess your claim. Many local authorities have implemented confidentiality procedures, and it is worth checking this with the Housing Department. The situation may be a good deal easier if your GP is aware of and sensitive to your worries about confidentiality.

If the local authority agrees to house you, you will probably be provided with temporary housing such as a hostel, bed and breakfast, or private rented premises while something more appropriate is found. Some local authorities in London also use what are called 'private sector leasing schemes', which are often Housing Associations who provide temporary flats for homeless people going through the Council.

If the authority does not accept that you are homeless, you will have to find your own accommodation. You can find out what options are available in your area through the local Housing Advice Centre, a Citizens Advice Bureau or a relevant voluntary organisation. The options are likely to include nightshelters, hostels, private flats, bedsits and bed and breakfast accommodation. There may also be housing projects or trusts that can help you.

These tend to be short-term options only. Nightshelters can be pretty grim, and offer only basic emergency accommodation to people with no money; they are not suitable for people who are ill. Bed and breakfasts are pricey, and good hostels with vacant rooms can be hard to find. To meet long-term housing needs, it would be a good idea to contact a Housing Advisory Service or a housing worker in an AIDS-specific organization.

Councils also operate their own housing system on a 'points' basis. In other words, a person applying to the Council for accommodation will be put down on the waiting list and awarded a number of points, depending on the Council's definition of need. People with HIV whose health is affected by their current housing conditions may receive a higher priority on the waiting list on medical grounds. You need a high number of points before you would even be considered for housing from the waiting list. In some areas, Council housing is so limited that even people with a high number of points have to wait a considerable period to be given accommodation. However, in some cases people with HIV illness may find that they can get housing more quickly from the Council on the points system, on the grounds that their accommodation is unsuitable for their needs and may be having a detrimental effect on their health.

Citizens Advice Bureaux, housing advice centres and other agencies listed in the Directory at the back of this book can provide further advice and guidance.

Harassment and Eviction

Harassment by a landlord may take a number of forms, such as violence, verbal abuse or threats, refusing to pay bills so that tenants have their gas and electricity cut off, and so on. People with HIV may be particularly vulnerable to harassment due to the ignorance and stigma that still surrounds the condition. Most tenants are legally protected from harassment, and from being evicted without the landlord going to court first. You will need to get further advice to find out what rights you have and whether you can stay permanently in your accommodation; many local authorities have a Tenancy Relations Officer who deals with issues between landlords and tenants.

If your situation has become particularly unpleasant and you want to leave, it is very important to make sure you get advice from a relevant agency. Leaving without finding alternative accommodation could place you in a very difficult position if you approach the local authority for housing and are considered to have made yourself 'intentionally homeless'.

Problems with Mortgage Repayments

If you are a home-owner with HIV and become ill, you may find it difficult to meet mortgage repayments if you are on sickness pay, or have had to resign from your job. It is important not to put off taking steps to deal with this possibility. You might qualify for Income Support (see *Financial Support*, above) in which case the DSS can help cover the interest payments on your mortgage. How much you receive will depend on the type of mortgage and the length of time it has been in existence.

If financial help is not forthcoming, and keeping the payments going is problematic, inform your bank or building society immediately. You may find that the loan can be renegotiated; most lenders are keen to reach an agreement which will enable the person involved to stay in the accommodation. Again, seeking further advice from relevant agencies may be useful.

Dealing with Employment Difficulties Related to HIV

The information in this section aims to offer you some guidance how to handle workplace discrimination; further advice should be available from your union and from legal agencies listed in the Directory at the back of this book.

Although employers cannot discriminate against job applicants on the grounds of gender, ethnic origin or marital status, there is no law to prevent them from refusing a job to someone who has HIV, is seen as 'high risk' for HIV, or cares for a person with HIV. If you feel you have been unfairly dismissed from a job you have held continuously for at least two years (or five years as a part-time worker), you have the right to present a claim for unfair dismissal to an industrial tribunal, unless you are in an organisation such as the police force or armed forces. (There is no qualifying period for claims of racial or sexual discrimination.) Taking a case to an industrial tribunal may seem gruelling, but even if you do not get your job back, you may obtain financial compensation or a reference.

Redundancy may occur if the company you work for is closing down or has changed in some way, so that your employer judges that there is no longer enough work for you to do. However, if you feel you have been made redundant for other reasons (for example your sexuality or HIV antibody status), or that your selection for redundancy differed from procedures established to make other redundancies, you may have a case for claiming unfair dismissal.

The Department of Employment's guidance on AIDS and the workplace states that being HIV positive is not grounds for dismissal. They have also recommended generally that employers of people whose health has declined so that they can no longer do the job they were hired for should find them alternative duties. Whether you can arrange this and the type of agreement you are able to make depend very much on the goodwill of your employer, since there is no legal obligation for alternative work to be found.

Getting Legal Help and Advice

You can get legal help from the organisations listed in the Directory at the back of this book; your local law centre or Citizens' Advice Bureau can help you find a sympathetic solicitor. You may also be eligible for legal aid to help with solicitors' fees.

Making a Will

This is not something most people think about until they get older or become ill. Making a will might appear to be an alarming step to take, because planning for death can raise some frightening issues. However it is important, because if you do not leave a will there are strict legal rules about the distribution of your possessions after your death. Making a will is not just about making sure money and property goes where we wish, but can cover funeral arrangements, appointing someone to look after your affairs when you die, and making sure dependent children have someone to look after them.

A will is a legal document, and although stationers now provide a 'do it yourself' form this is not recommended because if you write it yourself, it may contain legal ambiguities of which you are unaware. It is better to get a will drafted by a solicitor from private practice or from one of the organisations listed in the Directory at the back of this book. You may be eligible for legal advice and assistance.

Before getting advice about making a will, you need to think about what you own and to whom you wish to leave money or belongings. It is important to be aware that property or money held in joint names automatically passes to the survivor on death, regardless of the terms of a will. You also need to consider whom you would like as your *executor*. This is the person who looks after your affairs after you have died and carries out the wishes stated in your will. Pick someone you feel you can trust, and check that the person is happy about taking on this role.

It is possible to alter a will if you change your mind about any part of it. However, don't try and do this yourself: a separate legal document called a *codicil* is necessary and requires legal advice to be properly drawn up. Sometimes it is better to get a new will drafted instead. Remember to keep your will safe, and to let close friends or family know where it is.

Power of Attorney

A Power of Attorney is a document enabling one person to appoint another with the power to act on his or her behalf in financial and property matters. An ordinary Power of Attorney lapses if the person making it becomes mentally incapable. A person with HIV illness is advised to make an *Enduring Power of Attorney*, which will continue to be valid even if the individual becomes mentally incapable. An Enduring Power of Attorney must be registered at the Court of Protection. It may be a relief for you to feel confident that a trusted person has responsibility for financial decisions that might otherwise be a burden at times of crisis. It is important to remember that Power of Attorney confers no power to make medical or any other non-financial decisions on your behalf.

In much of Europe and the USA, 'Living Wills' or 'Advance Directives' set out a person's wishes regarding terminal medical care and are legally valid. They may also empower you to appoint someone to take medical decisions on your behalf. A 'Living Will' form for use by people with HIV and AIDS should shortly be available from the Terrence Higgins Trust.

Life Assurance and Mortgages

As mentioned in Chapter 6, if you have HIV, you will not be able to get life assurance, and should not apply for it. However, you may well be able to get a mortgage, even if you have been refused life assurance. There are two main types of mortgage: an endowment mortgage which requires life assurance and a repayment mortgage, which does not. In addition, there is an 'interest only' mortgage, which also does not require life assurance.

With a repayment mortgage, interest on the loan and the loan itself are paid back on a monthly basis. A repayment mortgage is generally available from a building society or mortgage broker, and if it does not involve life assurance, no information about your medical history, drug-injecting, sexual lifestyle, or your HIV antibody status is required. However, some lenders may require a 'mortgage protection policy'. This will depend on the amount of the loan and the ratio of the loan to the value of the property. A 'mortgage protection policy' is a form of life assurance, so a person with HIV will not be able to get one.

If you have applied for an endowment mortgage and your life assurance application is either refused by the insurance company or withdrawn by you, get in touch with the bank or building society to change your application to one for a repayment mortgage or an interest only mortgage. This may, however, mean accepting a smaller mortgage than might have been available with an endowment policy.

In a situation where you already have an endowment policy and are attempting to increase the loan on a property, do not surrender the policy. It can form part of the security for a new loan. Never exchange contracts on a property purchase until you are sure that all the financial arrangements are settled.

Organising a Funeral

Funerals, for the same reasons as wills, are often left to the last minute or forgotten altogether. It may seem strange to consider funeral arrangements when you feel well, or you may simply feel that your own funeral is not important. When and if you choose to plan your funeral at all is an entirely personal matter, and you may prefer to leave it to friends or family. On the other hand, you might feel that it is important that this memorable parting gesture should take place in the way that you would like, rather than the way others have decided for you.

Planning a funeral need not be a depressing affair. There is no need to stick to a religious service, unless this is what you would like. You can arrange whatever you want and can afford; readings from your favourite writers, music, singing, and so on. Your executor (see *Making a Will*, above) will need to know what your plans are, as he or she will be responsible for carrying them out. You might also want to talk this through with your family, or your partner.

Your funeral will be paid for with any money you leave. If you do not have enough, your executor or relatives will be asked to pay and, depending on their means, Social Security may cover some of the cost.

Coping with Being in Hospital

Going into hospital can provoke a range of responses in people, some of which may be hard to deal with. For some, being cared for in hospital can be a relief (at least temporarily), because it means being able to let other people look after them. For others it is exactly this sense of losing control over their lives that can be upsetting and disturbing.

How you feel about hospital care will depend on other factors, too. Cutbacks to the health service budget may mean staff have less time to spend on your care and limited resources to offer you. However, medical staff who are well trained in HIV issues are likely to provide a more sensitive service than those who are not.

If you have to go into hospital for a time, try to make it as productive as possible for yourself. Although it helps to get on well with your doctor, this does not mean you have to accept uncriticially everything he or she says. If you do not understand something, ask for clarification, and if you feel that something the doctor suggests may be inappropriate for you (or is inaccurate), don't be afraid to say so. Although many doctors are better informed and experienced in treating people with HIV illness than was true a few years ago, they do not always have all the answers. Challenging your doctor on any issue requires assertiveness and sensitivity, but it does not have to damage your relationship with him or her.

You may find having visitors in hospital supportive and encouraging or severely irritating. If you are tired or upset when you have a visitor with you, say so, or ask him or her to leave if necessary. You may be worried about hurting the person's feelings, but your visitor will probably understand that you have a lot to deal with at the moment. If not, it's really too bad - you have enough problems of your own to manage without taking on those of others.

Think about what you would like visitors to bring. You may find that if you are unhappy with hospital meals, food brought by visitors can be kept fresh for you in a fridge or oven in the hospital and supplement (or replace) meals provided. You may also like books, magazines, games, flowers, photographs, pens and paper, personal stereo and tapes, toiletries and so on. Sometimes the best present a visitor can bring you is news of outside events and gossip about people you know. If you're up to it, a good chat and a laugh can really lift your spirits.

You have the right to discharge yourself from hospital at any time, but this is a decision to be considered very carefully indeed. If you have complaints to make about the service you have received, make them clearly, as soon as you can, before making a decision to leave (see *Making a Complaint*, below). You may want to try another hospital if you think there is no means of improving your treatment, but the problem is that difficulties may arise if it is known that you discharged yourself from the first one. A local HIV/AIDS helpline or information agency could give you more help about hospitals providing good services for people with HIV.

Making a Complaint

Do not be afraid to complain if you feel you have been given inadequate or inappropriate service by people you deal with. If you don't, you may continue to receive poor treatment, and the situation could be repeated not just with you but with others in your position.

Medical Care

If you are unhappy with the care you are receiving, let the person caring for you know this. It is possible that your carer is underinformed about HIV illness, unsupported or overworked, and it may be possible to change this (certainly as far as awareness of HIV is concerned), or to reach an agreement that satisfies you both.

If the situation cannot be resolved through discussion, you can take the matter further. If your complaint is about professional conduct (for example, inappropriate disclosure of confidential information), you can pursue your complaint with the General Medical Council. This applies to all doctors, whether they are hospital doctors or GPs, NHS or private. If your complaint is about a dentist, whether private or NHS, contact the General Dental Council.

If your complaint is about poor service, the procedure depends upon whom you are complaining about. For complaints about NHS dentists and NHS GPs, you need to make a complaint to the Family Practitioners Committee. The procedure for complaining about NHS hospitals begins with the ward sister. If you need to take it further, complain to the house officer, registrar or consultant. If this is not satisfactory, take your complaint to the hospital administrator and/or the district administrator. As a last resort you can take the complaint to the Health Service Commissioner. *Whether your complaint is about NHS hospitals or GPs, enlist the support of the Community Health Council.*

It is also a good idea to inform your MP; this kind of action may help prevent the recurrence of negligence or bad practice related to HIV, and may raise general levels of awareness about appropriate care for people with HIV and AIDS.

Whatever your complaint, you need to be aware that there are time limits for making complaints which are different for different procedures. Contact an AIDS service organisation, law centre, advice centre or Citizen's Advice Bureau for more information about time limits.

Complaints procedures are not usually about obtaining compensation. If you are seeking damages for negligence, you will need to speak to a solicitor. You can contact advice and law centres for more information on how to proceed.

Blood and Organ Donation

If you have HIV, donating your blood, sperm, breastmilk or organs could put others at risk of infection. It is not a good idea to donate blood, organs and so on in order to find out whether you have HIV or not. You will not receive pre-test counselling, and a positive test result could be an unpleasant shock (see Chapter 6).

It is unethical for anybody to conduct an HIV antibody test upon your blood without your knowledge and consent. If a blood sample is taken from you, insist that you are informed about it, and give prior consent to any tests that could be carried out on it.

Vaccinations

Which vaccines to take and which to avoid are important questions for people with HIV. Views about which vaccines are safe tend to change quite regularly, so try to get the latest information from a doctor who is experienced in HIV issues. The points below are accurate at the time of writing, and should offer you some guidance.

- Vaccines which use inactivated virus, such as those for cholera, hepatitis B, diphtheria, tetanus and whooping cough are safe. However, repeated doses may be necessary for people with HIV because weakened immune systems may need a greater stimulus in order to begin producing antibodies.
- Department of Health guidelines state that live vaccines for rubella, measles, mumps and polio are safe for people who have

HIV. People with HIV illness can get an inactivated form of the polio vaccine.

- The BCG vaccine for tuberculosis should *not* be given to a person with HIV, and injections for yellow fever should not be given to a person with HIV illness.
- It is considered that most live vaccines apart from the BCG vaccine are safe for a baby with HIV, but it is a good idea to check with your doctor first, as he or she should be well acquainted with your child's state of health.
- Malaria tablets pose no risk to people with HIV, and neither does gamma globulin to protect against hepatitis A, since it is heat-treated.

Holidays and Travel Abroad

Organisations listed in the Directory at the back of this book can give you precise details about regulations and restrictions governing people with HIV and AIDS in different countries. You might also want to consider issues such as travel insurance, vaccination and immunisation, monitoring your health before you go away (see *Vaccinations* and *Keeping an Eye on Your Health*, above).

CLINICAL TRIALS OF DRUG TREATMENTS

Clinical trials of new drugs for HIV infection attempt to see how effective a treatment is, and how safe it is to use on people. The organisation of drug trials is a complex subject and one which tends to be off-puttingly riddled with jargon. The following section aims to give you basic information about trials, and suggests some of the questions you may need to ask if you are thinking of volunteering to join one.

Clinical trials of a new drug treatment are organised in three stages:

1. Phase one is designed to test a drug's safety;
2. Phase two tests how effective it is, and
3. Phase three compares it with other standard treatments already available.

A trial will recruit volunteers using strict entry criteria; the trial continues until specific 'end points' have been reached. These vary according to the state of health of those recruited in the trial, but some end points are fixed on the volunteers' eventual development of opportunistic infections or symptoms of immune suppression, or their death. The way in which a trial is set up and run is called its *protocol*.

Trials may last for months or even years in order to get a long-term view of the effects of a particular drug. Many involve the comparison of an experimental drug with a harmless substance, known as a *placebo*. As both the drug and the placebo look the same, volunteers will not know what they are getting, and neither will researchers (thus it is a *double-blind trial*). This is done to prevent the volunteers' expectations of getting better (if they know they are receiving the drug), or possibly worse (if they know they are receiving the placebo) from having any effect on the trial's results.

Since there is an obvious ethical difficulty about distributing placebos to people who might benefit from receiving drug treatment, some trials compare a new treatment with a standard drug that already exists, so that all volunteers involved are receiving treatment of some kind. Others may compare different dosage levels of the same drug, or give volunteers the option of whether to receive a placebo or not.

If a drug is finally judged to be successful, it may be given an official licence by the Committee for the Safety of Medicines at the Department of Health. However, even if a drug is unlicensed it may still be prescribed by doctors to specific patients on what is called a *named patient basis*.

Thinking about Joining a Clinical Trial

You might want further information about clinical drug trials in the UK, or you may be asked by a doctor or researcher whether you are interested in volunteering for one. If you are invited to join a trial, ask as many questions as you want about how it is run, how long it will last, what its aims are, any relevant information regarding the safety and efficacy of the drug concerned, and so on.

People have different reasons for participating in clinical trials. You may feel strongly that you want to help other people with HIV, or that joining a trial may be the only way for you to get access to a particular drug treatment. Whether you decide to enrol or not, make sure your decision is based on the best possible information available to you. Similarly, if you are looking for general information about drug trials in the UK, use as many different sources as you can. Apart from your doctor, there are local and national organisations which can provide further details (see the Directory at the back of this book).

One of the most important issues to consider is whether or not the trial has been approved by an ethical committee. Local ethical committees are made up of doctors and non-medical people, and have to decide whether a particular trial is ethically acceptable and scientifically necessary.

The fact that a trial has an ethical committee to oversee it does not, however, provide a guarantee that your best interests will be served by joining, but it may be unwise to think about joining a trial with *no* ethical committee, at least until you have got as much information about it as you possibly can.

If you do decide to enrol in a trial, new information about the drug involved should be given to you as soon as it is available. You have the right to leave the trial whenever you want, for whatever reason.

Some scientists and community organisations have become unhappy with the way clinical trials are designed and run. There are debates about issues such as the entry criteria to some trials, the length of time it takes for a drug to be licensed (if it ever gets to that stage), the degree of secrecy surrounding research of new drugs in the UK, and whether the basic rights of volunteers enrolled in trials are always considered and respected. Some of these issues are discussed further in Chapter 9.

CAMPAIGNING FOR CHANGE

Many aspects of living with HIV are likely to make you angry: media sensationalism and misinformation; other people's prejudice and complacency; discrimination in many different areas; uncertainty about the future; sometimes inadequate services and the fact that, despite all the money and time spent on medical research, there is still no vaccine or cure for HIV infection.

It can be hard to know what to do if you find you have powerful feelings of anger about coping with HIV. A possible solution may be to channel your anger into working for change. One way to confront this is to become involved with organisations campaigning to change attitudes and awareness of HIV and AIDS generally. Campaigning for change can take a number of forms: providing sensitive and accurate information and educational materials to journalists, policy-makers and the general public; doing careful public relations work, through parliamentary lobbying, setting up training programmes or taking part in face-to-face discussion and counselling. Change can also be enacted by means of direct action: expressing opposition to prejudice and unfair treatment by organising demonstrations, marches and rallies.

What and how much you are prepared to do depends on your free time, energy, skills and beliefs about effective campaigning measures. In addition to national and local organisations providing information, advice and help on HIV issues, some agencies now devote their resources entirely to pushing for basic rights for people with HIV infection (see the Directory at the back of this book).

8

CARING FOR A PERSON WITH HIV ILLNESS

Don't fall into the trap of thinking that 'caring for someone' means taking over someone's life and making decisions for them. Your real aim should be to ensure that it is possible for the person with HIV to live in the way he or she wishes.
 - *Caring for Someone with AIDS*, Research Institute for Consumer Affairs/Disabilities Study Unit

WHO CARES?

If you are caring for a person with HIV, you may be his or her lover, friend, acquaintance, relative, nurse, doctor, social worker, home help, health visitor - and so on. You may be paid to care, or you may not. Proper care for someone with HIV illness may involve a number of people offering widely varying degrees of help and support. Throughout this chapter the term 'carer' is used in its broadest possible sense. Issues confronting those carers looking after people with special needs such as women, children, drug users and people with haemophilia are dealt with in separate sections. You may also find it helpful to supplement the information given here with advice from organisations and publications listed in the Directory at the back of this book.

WHAT MAKES A GOOD CARER?

Generally speaking, there is no 'ideal carer'. Caring relationships vary; how much time and the kind of care you offer will depend on what is practical and manageable for you, and how close you are to the person with HIV. It may be helpful to ask yourself some of the questions below, if you are unsure what kind of care is appropriate (this will be of particular relevance to voluntary carers, but statutory workers with specific duties to fulfil may also find it useful).

- Who needs it? In other words, whose needs are you aiming to meet by offering care? Of course you are focussing on the needs of the person with HIV illness, but you may also have your own motivation. It could be, for example, that you want to provide care because it makes you feel useful, and wanted. It's fine to have your own needs for caring, but the needs of the person with HIV must come first.

- What is wanted? You may have ideas about the care you would like to offer, but this will be of little use to the person being cared for if, for example, someone else is already providing that support. Don't make assumptions about what help the person with HIV wants; ask. You might feel like having a good chat, but he or she might prefer you to do the housework. What you are able to offer will also depend on your skills and experience, and on what you feel comfortable with. The main thing is to enable the person being cared for to do what or she wants (but might not be able to cope with alone); caring is not about taking over another person's life.

- How much time should you spend caring? The crucial thing is to be realistic. You may feel a very strong desire to give as much help as you can if the person with HIV is a friend or a lover, but it is very important to take time to think this through before you make promises you cannot keep. You might be needed for a long period of time, and what seems manageable now could become increasingly demanding and tiring as time goes on. It is likely to be a big let-down for the person you are looking after if you make commitments now that you will not be able to carry out later. Try to work out exactly how much time and energy you can put into caring on a regular basis. It may be as little as an hour every week or so, or it may be far more. Remember that the time you spend can be flexible, depending on the needs of the person concerned. It is also helpful to have other people to take over from you from time to time, such as when you need a break or holiday.

- How will I get support? A carer who is exhausted and stressed is unable to be much use to the person being cared for. It is very important to check that you have people you can get help and support from, and ways of relaxing and unwinding. Your ability to provide care without becoming over-stretched may also be partly influenced by allowing yourself other interests. If you let caring for someone with HIV illness take over your entire life, the emotional strains it can impose could get the better of you. *Handling Burn-out* later in this chapter may be useful reading.

WHAT MAY CARING FOR A PERSON WITH HIV ILLNESS INVOLVE?

Fans of Florence Nightingale and hospital death-bed scenes might find it handy to read this section. Caring for someone with HIV illness may occasionally involve lightly dabbing cologne onto a fevered brow, but much of the time it could be a good deal more challenging and stressful than that. It is likely to include confronting uncertainty, prejudice and discrimination as well as the hardships caused by HIV-related illness itself.

People with HIV illness may have extremely wide-ranging needs, so carers could have a variety of demands to meet. Some of these are discussed below, and include providing information, offering practical help, listening to worries and anxieties and talking these through, handling financial difficulties, managing domestic problems, planning ahead, and so on.

Any carer who is looking after a person with HIV illness experiences the impact of HIV infection (even if at a distance) whether he or she is HIV negative or positive. Carers who are closely emotionally linked with the person they are caring for are likely to feel the stress of uncertainty discussed in the previous chapter, and may often feel as anxious or depressed as the person with HIV. In some cases, carers looking after people at a late stage of HIV disease may feel a strong sense of powerlessness, or even guilt because they themselves are healthy.

In addition to handling personal anxieties and concerns about the person's illness, a carer may also have to deal with his or her own feelings about illness. These can include anxiety, depression, panic and anger. None of these are easy emotions to deal with. In sexual relationships where one partner is caring for the other, the caring partner may be very worried about becoming HIV positive, even if safer sex is practised. If both partners are HIV positive, the caring partner may worry about getting ill and being unable to look after his or her lover.

There are other aspects of caring for a person with HIV illness that can be very hard to cope with, particularly if the carer is a close friend or lover. HIV can affect a person's brain and cause him or her to behave in uncharacteristic ways. Some of the more serious effects of HIV brain disease can be extremely upsetting. It may mean, for example, that the person concerned no longer recognises his or her carer; it may mean he or she becomes incontinent, or unable to communicate coherently.

However, HIV-related brain disease is very far from inevitable. More information on the subject is given in Chapter 2, but if you are concerned about how to cope should the person you care for become ill in this way, see the Directory at the back of this book for sources of help and support.

Finally, carers have to cope with the possibility that the person with HIV illness may die, despite everything that is done to help and support him or her. Death ~ our own and other people's ~ is something many of us are ill-prepared for. More information is given below in *Terminal Care, Death and Bereavement*.

STRATEGIES FOR CARE

Getting Involved

While many carers will be paid workers employed by social services and health authorities, there are also opportunities to work as a voluntary carer for organisations providing services for people with HIV. Details of specialist organisations of this sort are given in the Directory at the back of this book; in this chapter the role played by statutory carers is outlined below, under *Getting Help*.

Getting Information

One of the most practical ways you can help is by finding relevant information for the person you are caring for. It might help if he or she writes down a series of questions for you. Part of the research is likely to involve finding and contacting local agencies who can support, advise and offer practical help to you and the person with HIV (see the Directory). As research into HIV illness continues, there is a steady flow of information about new treatments and self-help measures. Sharing this type of news will not only keep the person you are caring for up to date, it may also help him or her stay positive about dealing with HIV illness.

You may find, if the person you are caring for is stressed or anxious, that you are asked the same questions more than once, because such feelings can make it hard to concentrate. It is quite likely that, for example, information passed on shortly after the time of diagnosis will not be retained very long – people are often in a state of shock when they first learn that they have HIV illness.

Being Honest

One of the most useful things you can do in a caring relationship is to be honest, to yourself as well as to the person you are looking after. This is easy to say, and often difficult to do. There will be times when you may feel hurt, exhausted, anxious, depressed or angry. It may seem that the easiest thing you can do is to ignore these feelings, so that you do not load your discomfort onto the person concerned. In some circumstances you may be right in thinking it inappropriate to discuss your feelings at length with the person you are caring for. After all, you are the carer and not the other way around. Whether you can or cannot do this will depend on his or her mental and physical state as well as the nature of your relationship.

If you are caring for a close friend or lover, it is possible that he or she may notice your mood anyway but feel unable to discuss it because you are keeping silent about it. In that situation, being honest about feelings you might regard as negative could well be the best move. Your friend might feel patronised if you insist that everything is fine, when it is obviously not. He or she may also feel worried that you are hiding dissatisfaction or anxieties; or may want to help. In any case, your feelings are unlikely to go away just because you pretend they do not exist, and the habit of struggling to appear all right can only add to any stress and anxiety you feel.

There are never any easy answers, but it may be the case that keeping quiet now about difficult issues may make it harder to say what is on your mind in future, even if you feel you really need to. Being honest about feelings is a subject on which a counsellor or carers' support group may be able to help and guide you (see the Directory).

If you are caring for someone on a more formal voluntary or paid basis, it could be a good idea to write your feelings down. As discussed in Chapter 7 this can help put them in perspective, since there are bound to be good days as well as bad. It can also help you develop ways of coping. Again, support and counselling could benefit you.

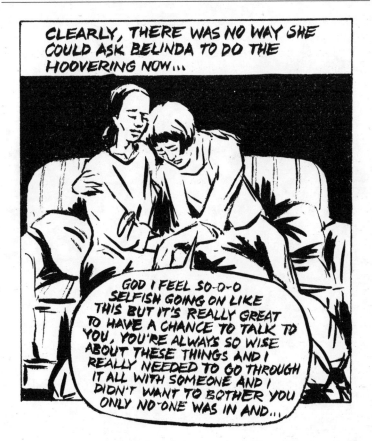

Above all, it may be comforting to remember that you do not have to be a saint to care for someone with HIV, in the same way that you would not expect this of the person you are caring for. If you feel angry or distressed as a direct result of something the person you are caring for has said or done, do not be afraid to say so. If you do not, he or she may behave in the same way again.

Sometimes the person with HIV may want to talk about his or her problems, but not know how to bring the subject up. On other occasions, he or she may feel that it is inappropriate to share them with you in case you then get depressed and anxious, particularly if you are a lover or a close friend. In such instances, don't pressurise the person into talking. It may help to say something fairly gentle like 'You seem upset/anxious/preoccupied. Is there any way I can help?' If the person with HIV does not want to talk, you cannot force him or her to do so. However, you may find that simple

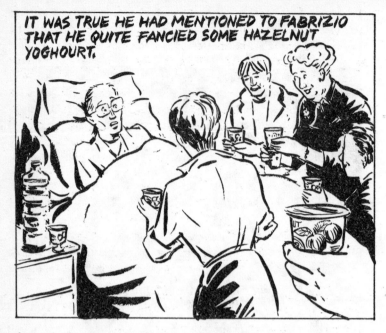

physical contact, such as holding hands, hugging, or sitting quietly together helps. It is often the case that just *being there* – the physical presence of a person who can be relied upon to provide support and not make judgements – is enough.

Above all, do not feel you have to keep a 'stiff upper lip'. Don't be reluctant to show that you care. If you feel like crying sometimes, then cry. If you feel moved to show physical affection through a kiss or a hug, do it. It might help to ask how the person concerned feels about this to begin with, if it is someone you don't know very well. People can feel swamped if you do not respect the limits they may want to set. Just saying 'I'd like to give you a hug. Is that all right?' should be enough. If the person *doesn't* want a hug, try not to take offence. He or she may simply not be in the mood, or not be particularly into hugging.

Ways of Caring

As stated earlier, the best way to find out what a person with HIV wants from you as a carer is to ask. The following suggestions may be helpful, but bear in mind that the needs of the person you are caring for may change.

- Phone up before you visit and check that the person wants to see you. It is important that the choice should be open. If the answer is no, don't take offence. He or she may feel tired and not like talking. Sometimes sending a card or ringing up to send best wishes can do as much good as a visit.
- When you do visit, bring things that will entertain, such as books, photos, magazines, tapes, records, and so on. Nice things to look at, such as flowers, plants, and posters may also be a good idea.
- Practical help around the home need not be limited to housework and shopping. If necessary, you could redecorate or re-arrange furniture – but ask first!
- Taking exercise – a walk, swim, cycle or run, for example – might feel good. How much exertion is possible will depend both on the state of health and frame of mind of the person with HIV. There is no point in undertaking an activity that is too strenuous and ends up causing exhaustion or depression because he or she no longer feels up to it.

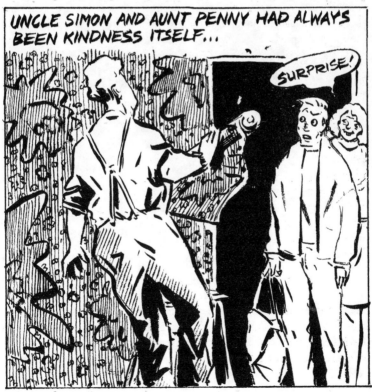

- Offer to cook a meal or to take the person out to a restaurant he or she is keen on.
- If the person has a young child (particularly if there is no partner to help), it is likely that he or she would be grateful for a babysitter from time to time. Help with changing nappies, bottle-feeding, and generally being around to play with the baby and keep an eye on him or her may also be appreciated.
- If the person feels well enough and enjoys dancing, why not go out to a club together? Apart from the exercise you get, there is also the pleasure of getting out and meeting old friends or new people. Remember that he or she may get tired quickly and want to go home earlier than you would like; it is important to respect this need.
- Assistance with writing letters, filling in forms and making phone calls that could cause stress or worry could be helpful. This could be related to work, finance, health care, social services ~ whatever. Make sure you ask for precise guidance first about the information that needs to be conveyed.
- Don't feel you have to be doing something constantly. He or she may just want to have you there to relax with, to watch television or a video perhaps. This can be as beneficial as any practical help. Providing gossip, jokes or funny stories can also be excellent ways of looking after someone ~ but make sure that the person you are caring for enjoys these, or you could find that they have the effect of a sleeping pill rather than a stimulant.

Avoid Judging

There may be times when you find you strongly disagree with the attitudes or beliefs held by the person you are caring for. Handling differences of opinion can be difficult, but it might help to remember that caring for someone with HIV does not mean you have to hide your point of view. If you disagree with what the person thinks or says, you are entitled to state this; pretending to agree when you do not could be patronising for the person concerned and stressful for you.

Whether and how you express disagreement is up to you, and a degree of sensitivity may be required to assess what is appropriate. In a very extreme case, you might feel that you are unable to develop a workable relationship with the person you care for. If it seems unlikely that talking through your concerns with him or her would be helpful, you could discuss them with a counsellor. It might be possible to sort out your difficulties, or it might not: sometimes caring relationships do collapse due to a clash of personalities. If that happens and you are not the only one involved in providing care for the person concerned, you might be able to find someone else to take over for you.

Stating differences of opinion is, however, not the same as expressing disapproval or condemnation of the person you care for. If you find you are constantly tempted to pass judgement on, for example, the sexuality, drug-taking habits or domestic arrangements of the person with HIV, you are not likely to be effective or helpful as a carer.

Handling Burn-out

'Burn-out' is the name given to a physical and mental state where you no longer feel able to cope with the duties of caring. You might be too exhausted, stressed, depressed, anxious or simply overwhelmed by a range of feelings to cope. Burn-out can be serious, and may have lasting effects, but if you recognise it and take a break or holiday when you need to, its impact can be temporary.

There is no universal solution to handling burn-out, other than to avoid it if you possibly can. Some of the suggestions given above will help: look after your health, don't take on more than you can provide on a regular basis, get other people to help you, have a break for a few days or weeks if you can manage this, and make sure you have friends, family, and/or a professional counsellor to support you. You need to be able to express the anger, frustration, grief, exhaustion or pain you may sometimes be feeling, as well as to share the pleasure and satisfaction caring can give. Take time to think about setting appropriate limits for yourself and about looking after your own needs.

Above all: treat yourself! Even if you're short of money, some treats ~ such as a cuddle, a hot foam bath, a massage, your favourite drink or meal, a walk in the country ~ can be arranged for free or reasonably cheaply. Looking after yourself can also mean taking time to rest, read, sleep, and be on your own for a while.

Getting Help

Don't try and take on the entire responsibility for caring. This could end up being exhausting and demoralising, which won't be good for you or the person being cared for. Whether you are a paid or unpaid carer, it is important to know what other help you and the person with HIV can get.

The range of services offering information, advice and practical help for people with HIV will vary from one region to another. The GP of the person for whom you are caring, the local authority social services, or an HIV/AIDS agency can give further details. Check with the person for whom you are caring as to what kinds of help would be useful, and whether he or she would prefer to contact the relevant service or have you do it.

Below, general health and social services that may be available in your area are discussed. In some cases, workers may have been trained specifically to care for people with HIV illness. Services set up to provide specialist care, and other useful organisations for people with HIV, are listed in the Directory at the back of this book.

Community Health Services

A GP is, in theory, a person's chief guide to health service options, and he or she will be crucial if the person you care for chooses medical care at home. In Chapter 4 some of the concerns relating to breach of confidentiality by GPs about HIV antibody status are discussed, and it is certainly the case that while some GPs are well-informed and sensitive regarding HIV issues, others are not.

A person with HIV can always change his or her GP, without having to give reasons for this. All that is necessary is to send the relevant medical card and a covering letter to the relevant Family Practitioner Committee. It is possible, however, that the new doctor will ask why the change was made.

You can get information about reliable GPs from friends, the local GU clinic, or local HIV helplines and support groups. There are also lists of local NHS GPs' surgery hours and appointment systems kept in the office of the Community Health Council (District Council in Northern Ireland, Local Health Council in Scotland), in the post office, libraries and Citizens Advice Bureaux.

It may help to remember that people can get care at home without a GP. Some of the options are discussed below (where they are linked to a general practice, this is indicated); other organisations specialising in providing home care for people with HIV are listed in the Directory at the back of this book.

Health Visitors

Health visitors are nurses who give advice on staying healthy and coping with the practical aspects of being ill at home. They are likely to be able to provide you with a lot of information about other services available locally. They can also advise on emotional problems such as dealing with stress, anxiety and depression.

District Nurses

District nurses are trained to care for people at home and are attached to a general practice, so a person with HIV who is not registered with a GP would find it difficult to get help from one. The service provided is wide-ranging, covering tasks such as bathing, administering dressings, giving injections and so on. They can train carers to carry out such tasks, and can also give advice on coping with other issues, such as dealing with bed sores or problems moving around.

A district nurse may also be able to arrange special equipment such as walking frames or bathing aids, and can contact local voluntary agencies or social services for you, if required.

Macmillan Nurses

Macmillan nurses were originally appointed to care for people with cancer but may, in some health districts, also help people with other diseases that are considered incurable. They are senior nurses who are trained to help and advise on patient care and dealing with the practical as well as the emotional aspects of illness. They are also trained to provide counselling. A GP, local hospital or district nurse can tell you about the Macmillan nursing team in your health district.

Community Psychiatric Nurses

CPNs are trained to help people with emotional problems, such as prolonged depression relating to illness. They provide advice and assistance at home, and may either be able to offer counselling themselves or will refer you to a local agency that can provide this.

Physiotherapists

Physiotherapists can visit at home, but some are based in hospitals. Their role is to help patients develop muscular strength and movement, and they could help a person with HIV be as active as possible.

Occupational Therapists

Occupational therapists are there to help people who might be too ill to carry out day-to-day tasks such as bathing, dressing and eating. Their services are based on showing people new ways to do the things they may have difficulties with, and by providing equipment such as wheelchairs, bath seats or raised toilet seats. Occupational therapists work from hospitals and social services departments.

Social Services

Social workers, who can offer help and support for someone living at home with HIV or AIDS, are trained to advise on wide-ranging emotional, practical and financial issues, and are mainly based in the social services departments of local authorities. There are also social workers based at hospitals who may take charge of organising home care, and in some areas workers have a special responsibility for looking after people with HIV, AIDS and their carers (see the Directory for details).

Above all, social workers can put you in touch with other sources of practical help in the community. These could include *home helps*, who are employed by social services departments and can do domestic tasks such as laundry, shopping and housework. If preparing meals is a difficulty, *Meals on Wheels* can deliver hot food on a regular basis, and, if you live in the Greater London area, *The Food Chain* organisation will deliver nutritious three-course meals for free (social services departments and HIV agencies can give you further details). Some social services departments run a laundry service, which although mainly for people who are incontinent could also accept laundry from people who are not well enough to do their own washing. In addition, you may be able to get help from an occupational therapist (see above).

Counselling

In Chapter 6 the significance of counselling before and after an HIV antibody test is discussed. Counselling may also be of benefit to people with HIV and their carers at other times. A good counsellor is a person who does not judge you, tell you what you should do, or impose his or her own views upon you. He or she can, however, help you to recognise the difficulties you have to deal with and support you in finding ways of doing so.

Counselling techniques vary, as do costs. There may be no charge at all, a nominal fee, or a sliding scale of charges depending on the income of the client. However, you must be able to expect complete confidentiality, and if you are uncertain about this, check that the counsellor understands that this is vital. Also feel free to ask whatever questions you wish about the counsellor's training and techniques. It is up to you to make sure that you find the right person for you, even though this may not become clear until you have had a number of sessions. If for any reason you decide not to continue with counselling, there is no obligation to do so. The terms of agreement between you and the counsellor are generally discussed in the first session.

Counselling can be a demanding process, as quite often it involves looking at situations which have caused you anger and distress. It is possible that you may feel worse before you feel better, as you begin to confront hidden feelings. It is worth bearing in mind that you are likely to feel better ultimately and that although you may sometimes feel that you are making no progress, getting back in touch with buried emotions and learning from them is, in itself, positive.

National organisations have counsellors trained and experienced in HIV-related issues, and local HIV, gay and lesbian helplines and support groups may provide counsellors on HIV and AIDS (see the Directory for details).

Specialist HIV Services

Specialist services for people with HIV in the community may be offered by national and local organisations. If you are uncertain about what is available in your area, a national HIV agency can give you more information.

The range of services set up to help people with HIV include:

- Helplines
- Face-to-face counselling
- Support groups (sometimes these are available to carers as well as to people with HIV)
- Day centres
- Drop-in centres
- Respite care (looking after a person with HIV who has recovered from a recent illness but does not feel well enough to return home)
- Buddies (trained volunteers who look after people with HIV illness, and can also offer support to partners, friends and family)
- Home support teams
- Legal and financial advice
- Information, health education, and resource centres (sometimes these also provide literature in languages other than English)

What is available to you in your area will depend largely on how the relevant health and local authorities view HIV infection. It remains the case that health districts which record a relatively large number of people with AIDS in their area tend to be better provided with services than those which do not. Information about the range of services offered by major HIV organisations and other associated agencies is given in the Directory at the back of this book.

CARING FOR A CHILD WITH HIV INFECTION

If you are caring for a child with HIV you may find you are constantly worrying about the child's health, and anxiously checking for signs of illness. As discussed in Chapter 2 (which gives more information about symptoms of illness, and treatments for children with HIV), the survival time of a baby or young child with HIV is generally less than that of an adult.

This is partly because the child's immune system may not be as well-developed and able to cope with infection. However, it is broadly true that children who survive the first year or so of HIV infection without symptoms of illness have a better chance of living well with HIV than children who become ill within a matter of months after birth.

Looking after a child with HIV may be particularly demanding for other reasons. A child who is too young to talk cannot use words to tell you his or her needs and how to fulfil them, which in infants who are often ill may be particularly frustrating and upsetting. You are likely to find that the child's body language and crying can tell you a great deal, and that your own intuition and sensitivity will be of considerable help. Often, basic needs for reassurance and comfort can be met by cuddling, rocking, talking to and holding the child. However, if he or she is ill it is important to get medical attention; do not try and interpret symptoms of illness on your own. Although many children with HIV disease have complaints which are common in HIV-negative children, more serious illness can be prevented if a doctor is able to treat infections at an early stage.

In general, it is safe to give children with HIV live vaccines, although the BCG vaccine for TB should not be given (see Chapter 7).

Discussing HIV with a Child

It may often be very distressing to look after a child with HIV, because the child may not understand why he or she is ill, and may feel frightened as well as sick. If you are the child's parent, you are very likely to be the first person he or she turns to for comfort and support. With a child who is old enough to talk, that may mean tackling some difficult questions. Some of these may put you at a loss because you do not want to frighten the child with ideas about death, or you may just not know the answers.

There are differing views about what and how much to tell a child about having HIV infection. Perhaps the key points to consider are that it helps if the child feels comfortable with the person who gives the information, which must be presented with care and sensitivity, using words and images that the child can understand. It may, for example, help to think up games that help get the information across. Sometimes pictures can present ideas more clearly than words to young children. Care and sensitivity are essential because the information needs to be communicated in as relaxed and unintimidating a way as you can possibly manage. For example, you may feel that it is not a good idea to bring up the subject of death, which many young children have difficulty grasping (as do adults). Most children, on the other hand, are able to understand what illness is.

Having up-to-date information will help you, because you will then be able to give accurate answers to as many questions as you feel to be appropriate. It will also help you to feel in control and to keep the child's HIV infection in perspective. This is particularly important when new drug treatments for infections in children with HIV are becoming increasingly available, and research into use of anti-viral drugs such as zidovudine is likely to lead to therapies that can help limit damage to the immune system (see Chapter 3). Ways of testing for HIV that will allow an early diagnosis in young children are also likely to become more widely available in the near future.

There is no need to feel that you have to cover every aspect of HIV infection at one sitting with the child for whom you are caring. It may help to see the process as an ongoing dialogue, with the child able to feel he or she can ask more questions later on. If you don't know the answer to any of these, it is probably best to say so. It will help if the child feels that he or she can trust you to be honest, and can rely on the information you give. It is also important that he or she has all the time and encouragement needed to talk about fears and unhappiness. This may be painful to cope with, but it could be more problematic in the long run if the child feels he or she should not discuss being afraid or sad, in case you are upset by this. Children can be very good at protecting loved ones from difficult emotions, very often at their own expense.

Coping with Feelings of Guilt or Regret

If you are a parent caring for a child with HIV, it may be hard for you to avoid feeling guilty or responsible in some way for the child's infection. Mothers with HIV sometimes report feeling extreme distress and guilt when their babies have tested HIV antibody positive. Men with HIV who have passed the virus to their female partners when having unprotected sex in order to have children may experience similar feelings, particularly if the baby also turns out to be HIV positive.

Guilt and regret are very tough emotions to deal with, and you may want to get help from a counsellor and/or support group for carers. Talking to other people in a similar situation is likely to help, as is being able to vent your distress with a neutral person who can listen and give support.

It may help to remember that very few (if any) people with HIV have any desire to pass the virus on to others. The image of HIV-positive people as irresponsible maniacs whose main aim in life is to infect as many others as possible is purely sensationalist nonsense; unfortunately such rubbish still serves to sell newspapers. You did not choose for the child you care for to be HIV positive, and you would not have wished it. You are no doubt doing the very best you can to manage a situation which can sometimes be distressing and demanding. Blaming and feeling bad about yourself is inappropriate, and may also make it difficult for you to provide the care and support your child will need, and to get help and support yourself.

Telling Other People

Children, like adults, can suffer stigma and abuse as a result of other people knowing that they have HIV infection. The two key questions to ask before you tell anyone about the child's HIV antibody status are: Who has the right to know? and Who needs to know?

It is possible that no one has the *right* to know. However, people like the child's GP or health visitor may need to know, if not knowing will prevent them from providing proper care and treatment for the child, or support for you.

You may also feel that there are people you would like to tell.

However, the effects of telling people about the child's HIV antibody status could be serious if they do not respond in the way you anticipate, or do not keep the information to themselves (see Chapter 7). Friends who seemed reliable may prevent their children from having contact with the child once his or her antibody status is known – in some cases a child's entire family has been ostracised by other people. It may be a good idea to speak to a counsellor if you have doubts or worries about what to do. It might also help to gather as much information as you can to answer the possible questions and concerns of people you decide to tell.

If you are the parent or foster parent of a child with HIV, there is no obligation to tell the child's babysitter or minder. Good hygienic practice, which is adequate to prevent HIV transmission, should be followed in any case. However, it may help to weigh up factors such as the potential difficulty of the childminder finding out a later stage, if your child begins to become ill.

Similarly, there is no obligation for staff, parents or children involved with playgroups, nurseries or schools to be informed, for the same reasons. The most important motivation for telling a member of staff would probably be if the child were likely to receive more sensitive care and attention as a result. Such decisions need very careful consideration.

Preventing HIV Transmission

There is no need to take special precautions to prevent a child with HIV passing the virus to others. As stated earlier in this book, HIV cannot be transmitted through ordinary social contact. Ordinary hygienic precautions outlined under *Taking Care at Home* in Chapter 7 are quite adequate to prevent viral transmission. Heavily soiled clothing can be dealt with in the hot cycle of a washing machine, while using disposable nappies for a young child with HIV may make life easier for you (although they are more expensive than washable ones, and some people object to them on environmental grounds). There is no risk of HIV infection through changing nappies, but simple measures such as washing your hands after each nappy change (especially before handling food) and keeping cuts on your hands covered with sticking plaster are sensible measures to prevent other infections, such as hepatitis and salmonella, developing as a result of contact with faeces.

If the child has an accident involving spilled blood, hot water and bleach (preferably in a ratio of ten parts water to one part bleach) are adequate to clean it up. Wearing disposable latex gloves to clean up blood spillages will further reduce any risks of HIV infection from the child's blood, although some carers may feel uncomfortable about doing this, in case the child feels stigmatised. It may help to remember that good hygienic practice should be followed for *all* children where possible, not just for those who are known to have HIV infection. This is the safest and most sensible way to prevent HIV transmission through accidents involving spilled blood; it is also the least discriminatory.

Children with HIV infection should be able to lead as normal a life as possible. This means going to school, making friends and playing with other children. Taking part in sports, sharing wind instruments or getting involved in other social and group activities at school do not present a risk to other children. Activities which involve the potential exchange of blood, such as becoming 'blood' brothers and sisters (where blood is shared as a type of bond between people) are risky, however. Similarly, sharing equipment to inject drugs is extremely risky; Chapter 4 looks at drug-use issues in more detail.

In general, it is more likely that a child with HIV will be at risk of illness from other children than vice versa. For this reason, you might want to keep a child with HIV away from school for a time if there is an epidemic of flu or chickenpox, for example.

If the child you are caring for is of an age to be interested in and thinking about sex, he or she will need clear information about how HIV is transmitted and how to have safer sex. It can be very hard on young people with HIV to find out that they have a sexually transmitted disease before they have really begun to understand their sexuality and developing sexual relationships.

Sex is one subject many parents find difficult enough to discuss with adults of their own age, let alone with their children. However, it is important for any young person, whether living with HIV or not, to be given clear, non-judgemental messages about safer sex in language he or she can understand and will not find intimidating. It also helps to make information about safer sex positive and encouraging; presenting it as a set of restrictions rather than possibilities is likely to be very demotivating. If you are in a close caring relationship with a young person who has HIV (for example, as a parent or foster parent) you might want to talk to them about safer sex. What and how to talk about it may seem like a major worry, but you can get help from some of the useful organisations and publications listed in the Directory at the back of this book.

Chapter 5 of this book may be useful reading, although you may need to judge how much detail to provide if the young person is at an early stage of sexual awareness and might be confused by too much information at once.

TERMINAL CARE, DEATH AND BEREAVEMENT

Terminal Care

Caring for a terminally ill person may well be exhausting, frustrating and very distressing. You might feel that you just don't know what to say to comfort the person you are caring for. It doesn't matter if you are sometimes stuck for words: just being around to listen, or holding hands in silence could be all that's needed. The physical presence of someone who is trusted and familiar can sometimes have a much more reassuring effect than words can ever have.

Care of a dying person, or terminal care, may take place in hospital, in a hospice, or at home. The most appropriate option will be determined by what the person concerned wants and needs, and by what is available locally. Such decisions are not always easy to make, and may need to involve a good deal of thought. The following section gives brief information about options for terminal care.

At Home

Being cared for at home, where you feel most comfortable and can have your own things around you, is an option many terminally ill people prefer. Successful terminal care at home depends on the medical condition of the person concerned; in some cases it may not be feasible because needs such as pain relief, which can require specialised nursing, may not be adequately met. It may also be difficult if the person being cared for lives alone, as local services may not be sufficiently comprehensive to provide the continuous attention required.

In other cases, the provision of basic equipment (such as a wheelchair, bathseat, or handrails by the bed or toilet) to make life comfortable for the person with HIV is adequate to create an appropriate environment for home care. You will need to contact the occupational therapist attached to the relevant hospital or homecare team for more information about this. If you are caring for a terminally ill person with HIV at home, you must make sure that you have all the help you can get from local health and social services as well as relevant voluntary agencies.

Hospices

These are set up to look after people with an incurable disease, who may be too ill to be cared for at home and who may no longer respond to medical treatments. Standards of care in many hospices are very high; staff are generally specially trained to meet patients' emotional needs as well as providing relief from pain. They generally allow visitors throughout the day and night, and may also provide support for family and friends during bereavement.

Hospices tend to be run in different ways, and their admission criteria vary. Many are run by voluntary organisations or charities, although some are funded by the NHS; the majority do not charge patients. You can get more information on hospice care generally and details of the one nearest to you from your GP, social worker or Citizens Advice Bureau. The local library should also have details. People can apply to a hospice directly, or through health or social workers.

There are still few hospices specifically for people with HIV in Britain; see the Directory for details.

Hospital

For some people, dying in hospital might appear to be the least attractive option. Hospitals can be intimidating places, where people may feel a lack of privacy or control over what is happening to them. However, because of the specialised nature of the care a terminally ill person may require, home or hospice care may not be appropriate. Medical staff who have been trained to provide care for people with HIV illness should be well equipped to make sure that the person concerned has everything he or she wants, and is made as comfortable as possible.

Feelings about Death

While writing this chapter I was told that two men with AIDS I came to know through working at the Terrence Higgins Trust had died. Though neither was a close friend, I was fond of them both. Although I was not involved in caring for either Simon or Danny, their deaths fill me now with a mixture of grief and anger. That two young men who had so much to offer and had already given so much should now be dead seems an outrage, the most senseless waste of human life. I miss them, and I want them back.

Death is a reality which many of us look at through a screen of embarrassment and fear, not wanting or unable to find words to discuss its impact upon our lives. We tend to understand it so badly, and give ourselves little time and space to come to terms with our feelings of grief and loss.

The process of bereavement is, however, often one which begins *before* someone has died. Carers may have to face that the person they are looking after is ready for death and has come to terms with it, when they themselves have not. At such times, the first instinct of the carer may be to silence discussion about dying, in order to stamp on what he or she may regard as 'morbid thoughts'. Unfortunately, you may find that silence or an enforced jollity are only likely to distance you from the person you are caring for.

Women and men with HIV illness may want to talk about death for various reasons – because, like most people, they are frightened of the idea and do not know what to expect, or perhaps because they are ready to face it and want to think about making practical arrangements, such as organising their funeral. A person with HIV who seems reasonably well but wants to talk about death should not be treated as a depressive, someone who is taking a grimly pessimistic view of manageable circumstances. Even if death seems a long way away for both you and the person you are caring for, if he or she wants to talk about it then it is a good idea to do so. Discussion of death does not necessarily mean that the person who raises it has 'given up' on life: it could simply mean that he or she wants to be prepared and plan ahead.

Another reason why it might be unhelpful to avoid discussing death with the person you are caring for is that the person with HIV illness can slip into the role of 'comforter' for you by not discussing subjects that he or she feels are likely to upset you. This is particularly hard on someone who is seriously ill.

It may help if you can make clear at an early stage of the relationship that the person concerned is free to talk with you about whatever is on his or her mind. That means that the person with HIV can take the initiative and raise the subject if he or she wishes to do so. This will require tact and sensitivity. However, discussing death may be easier to manage if it has taken place over a period of time in a reasonably relaxed manner, rather than right at what may feel like the last minute.

What to Do When Someone Dies

Having to handle practical arrangements relating to death can make life harder just at a time when you are trying to cope with the trauma of loss. If you are responsible for handling practicalities such as the financial affairs of the person who has died, funeral arrangements and registration of the death, get as much support and help as you can from friends, family and relevant HIV organisations. You should also find that the people you deal with - the funeral director, registrar, and so on - can explain what is necessary and give you guidance.

A Death at Home

When someone dies, his or her doctor needs to be informed at once. He or she will complete a *death certificate* giving the cause of death, so that it can be registered. If the body is to be cremated, the doctor will need to know this, as he or she will have to examine it, as will a second doctor.

A funeral director will either remove the body or lay it out so that other people can come and say goodbye. Laying out the body involves stopping up bodily orifices, tidying and dressing it. This can be upsetting, particularly if the funeral director opts to wear protective clothing, which some prefer to do.

A Death in Hospital

If the person has died in hospital, a hospital doctor will issue the death certificate, stating the cause of death. This may be given as the immediate cause, i.e. the relevant opportunistic infection, rather than HIV illness or AIDS. If it will be a problem for HIV illness to be mentioned as the cause of death (for example, if the person who has died did not tell family members his or her HIV antibody status, and would not have wished them to know), it is important to discuss this with the doctor. He or she may be prepared to list the infections responsible for death without mentioning HIV, or may agree to confine the information about HIV to a separate letter to the Registrar.

The funeral director can be given authorisation by the person's executor or a relative to take the body away from the hospital mortuary.

Registering the Death

The death certificate will need to be taken to the Registrar for the area where the death occurred. In England and Wales, this must generally be done within five days of the death; in Scotland it is eight days. You can find details of local registrars of births and deaths in doctors' surgeries, post offices and public libraries.

Once a death is registered, a document known as the *disposal certificate* is given, without which burials or cremations cannot take place. You will also need certified copies of the entry of death in the register for purposes such as claiming life assurance, National Insurance or Social Security benefits. The Registrar can give you these, and explain to you what they are for.

Coroners

If the person who has died was not seen by a doctor during their last illness or if the doctor certifying death did not see the person during the last 14 days of illness, or following the death, a coroner will have to be informed of the death. A death will also need to be reported to a coroner if there are suspicious circumstances or if the death was due to unnatural or unknown causes. The coroner may decide to arrange a post-mortem examination, and if the cause of death remains uncertain or is considered in doubt or unnatural, to hold an inquest.

Organising the Funeral

As stated in Chapter 7, funeral arrangements can be included in a person's will, but they are not legally binding. It is generally up to the executor, or next of kin if there is no will, to plan the funeral.

Funeral directors can organise the burial or cremation, and will also explain any forms you may need to complete and fees that are payable. The relevant trade association is called the National Association of Funeral Directors, and it should provide details of services and prices, with a written estimate of what any particular funeral will cost.

Sometimes you can get help from your local authority with organising a funeral. Some may provide a municipal funeral service, which will probably be cheaper than organising the funeral privately. Others may be able to help pay for it if you or others do not have the funds to do so. You will need to contact the local authority Social Services or Environmental Health Department to find out if this is possible. Remember that there is no need to have a religious service, unless this is what the person asked for.

For cremation to take place, the cause of death must be established. The death will have to be registered and a registrar's or coroner's certificate issued. There are a number of forms to be filled in for a cremation to be properly authorised – these can be obtained from a funeral director (who can explain them to you) or from the crematorium. You may want to keep the cremated remains after the service. It should be possible to make arrangements to do this with the funeral director or crematorium.

Coping with Bereavement

Even if you feel reasonably well prepared for the death of someone you have been caring for, it is never easy to be sure how you will respond to it when it actually happens.

Bereavement can give rise to feelings which might sometimes seem difficult and inappropriate. You may, for example, feel numb and detached, shocked, acutely distressed, unable to accept the reality of death, confused, frustrated or desperate. You may also sometimes feel relief, a strong sense of love and sexual desire, anger at being 'left behind', or guilt about things you said or did (or did not say or do). If you are HIV positive, the death of a person with HIV illness may cause you distress and anxiety about your own future. Carers who have to cope with a number of friends dying from HIV illness might find the burden of repeated loss very hard to bear.

Try not to be afraid of these feelings, nor of talking them through with other people. If you are able to talk to your friends, lover or family, that can be enormously helpful. There are also counsellors, helplines and support groups to help you cope. It is important that you share your grief and look after you own needs during this very difficult time.

For a carer who has experienced bereavement, one of the hardest feelings to cope with is the sense that grief is somehow embarrassing or difficult for others. Another is the idea that grieving is appropriate only for a set period of time, after which you must develop a 'stiff upper lip' and get on with your life. For these reasons mourning the death of someone you were close to can be an intensely lonely experience, although it does not need to be.

If you can, it may help to spend time with someone else who knew the person who has died. Being with other people who are going through bereavement can be a relief, making it easier for you to share your feelings of loss and grief. It can be very reassuring to know that there are other people who understand a bit about what you are going through. You may also find that you are desperate to talk about the person who has died with another person who knew him or her; this can be very helpful in getting through bereavement.

Unfortunately, you might find that people want to 'help' you get over your feelings by silencing discussion about them. This is not the kind of help you need. Sometimes other people find grief awkward and delicate, regarding it as something to keep quiet about. It is not. Grieving is a natural and essential part of saying goodbye to someone and showing your appreciation of him or her. If people try to persuade you to 'put on a brave face', ignore them. Keeping your feelings to yourself may make life a little easier for them, but it is unlikely to do so for you.

There is no prescribed period of time necessary to get over the pain and loss of death. It is likely to take quite a long time, but may be harder and more prolonged if you do not allow your feelings to come to the surface and be acknowledged; by crying, screaming, talking or whatever you feel like doing, you are beginning the process of healing and recovery.

Remembering the good times you had with the person who has died may be traumatic if the last few weeks or months were clouded by his or her illness and pain. However, those times were real and cannot be taken away from you. Looking at photographs and letters, or reading through diary entries about happier times may be acutely upsetting now, but when you are ready they will provide you with an important record of what you shared. If you find the memories too painful for the time being, do not rush yourself. There will be a time when they bring you pleasure again.

Looking Ahead

In the short term, living with bereavement may mean asking for time off work for compassionate reasons. You may need your GP or hospital to back you up on this. It might help to think of grieving as a process involving different stages, beginning with shock and working through denial, anger and loss to acceptance. Although there is no hard and fast rule as to the pattern of emotions connected with bereavement, your pain will lessen with time and it is likely that the memories of happy rather than unhappy times with the person you cared for will be the longest-lasting ones.

In the long term, you may find other ways of helping yourself through the grieving process. One is to get involved with a project in memory of your friend. You may want to do this on your own or with friends, and it could involve (for example) expressing your feelings and memories through creative work – such as writing, painting or drawing – dedicated to the person you cared for. What

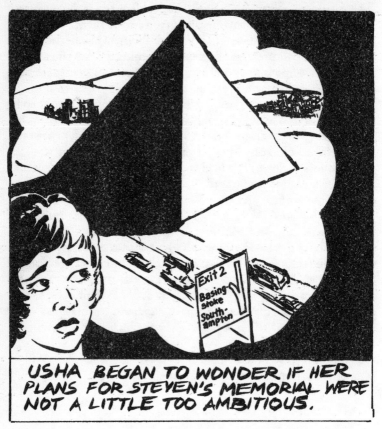

USHA BEGAN TO WONDER IF HER PLANS FOR STEVEN'S MEMORIAL WERE NOT A LITTLE TOO AMBITIOUS.

you decide to do is obviously a matter of your interests and skills, but it may help to speak to other carers who have looked after someone who has died; they might give you some ideas and further information.

One memorial project for people with HIV that now has an international reputation is the *Names Project Quilt*. This is an enormous quilt made up of memorial panels sewn by the friends, lovers and families of people who have died with HIV illness. Although the idea originated in the United States, panels in the quilt are now from countries all over the world, including Britain. There are now over 4,000 panels, and pieces of the quilt have been exhibited internationally. If you would like to get involved with making a panel to commemorate a person who has died with HIV illness, details of how to contact the *Names Project UK* are given in the Directory at the back of this book.

This chapter has emphasised the importance of allowing yourself to acknowledge and express the powerful feelings that might arise from caring for a person with HIV illness. One of the most forceful of these may be anger, particularly if you have experienced the prejudice and hostility that some people feel towards people with HIV and their carers.

Anger can be frightening, particularly if you sometimes feel unsure of how to channel it or what causes it. However, as stated in Chapter 7 anger can be a source of energy and a powerful motivating force. If you are unhappy about any aspect of the care the person you were looking after received, or about public awareness of HIV generally, you may want to direct your dissatisfaction into working for change. Many organisations providing services for people with HIV employ a large number of volunteers as well as some paid workers. What you are prepared or able to do will depend on your skills, experience and interests, but organisations listed in the Directory may give you some ideas about services that could benefit from your input.

9

CRUCIBLE OF THE FUTURE

AIDS is a crucible in which the future of health is being forged.
– *Jonathan Mann, former head of the World Health Organization's Global Program on AIDS*

According to Dr Jonathan Mann the world has been affected by HIV through three separate epidemics. Dr Mann identified the first epidemic as that of HIV, a largely invisible spread of infection which may have begun in the 1950s or 1960s. The second is a steady increase in people with AIDS world-wide. The third is made up of the denial, delays in organising relevant services, and discriminatory measures against people who are HIV positive (or assumed to be so) that have characterised the response on the part of many countries to HIV and AIDS.

By April 1991, the official WHO estimate for global cases of HIV was between 10 and 15 million, and a cumulative total of 345,533 people with AIDS had been recorded, a figure considered to be under-reported by as much as 50 per cent. For those who have become casualties of Mann's third epidemic of discrimination, there are no available statistics. This chapter looks at discriminatory measures against people with HIV in detail.

Other than Antarctica, there is now no continent that is unaffected by all three epidemics. As stated earlier in this book, the fact that HIV and AIDS are linked with the powerful taboos of sexual behaviour and drug use may go some way to explaining why many governments have wasted years either ignoring the need to take action or insisting that it was a matter for other people, other countries to worry about. Perhaps this is also why some scientists have been preoccupied less with the rate and route of spread of the virus than with a search for its origin, a process which has often involved some highly dubious research.

BACK TO THE BEGINNING

Theories that AIDS started in Africa are based on the idea that HIV is a mutation of a virus known to affect African monkeys – the Simian (monkey) Immunodeficiency Virus, or SIV. In June 1989, links were shown between a strain of HIV called HIV2 and a type of SIV found in wild sooty mangabeys in West Africa. Similarly, less significant genetic links have been established between HIV and another form of SIV discovered in green monkeys in Central Africa. This research has been interpreted as showing that HIV viruses have been transmitted from animals to humans within the past 20 to 40 years. It does not, however, explain how or where transmission could have occurred, although there has been speculation about bizarre sexual practices involving monkeys. If HIV is a mutation of SIV (and there is no clear evidence of this), it is more likely to have become so through contact between monkeys and humans in the laboratory, where SIV was first identified, than through sexual practice. The idea that HIV came from Africa has never been properly proven; it remains the product of inadequate research and racism.

Similarly, an early idea that AIDS began in Haiti was shown to be the result of irresponsible speculation. It stemmed from confusion over the existence of heterosexual Haitians with AIDS when in the United States the condition was regarded as only affecting gay men. However, as the AIDS epidemics in Haiti and the United States were more or less simultaneous, the theory had to be abandoned.

There is also no reliable evidence that AIDS is the outcome of germ warfare experiments by the KGB or the CIA (to which agency it is attributed depends more on political leaning than on hard information), nor that it is the result of inadequate sterilisation of gamma globulin used to treat hepatitis in gay men in the 1970s, nor that it came from outer space, as was suggested by a British scientist in 1986. Attempts to interpret the condition as a heaven-sent device to purge the earth of so-called 'undesirable groups' such as gay men or injecting drug users are easily discredited by the fact that non-injecting heterosexuals become infected.

By far the vast majority of scientists and doctors now regard HIV as the cause of AIDS – this was not the case initially because HIV was not identified until 1983. However since, as stated in Chapter 1, AIDS (or GRIDS, as it was then called) was associated with gay men in the US when it was first apparent, early research linked it with factors seen to be common to a 'gay lifestyle'. These included sniffing amyl nitrate (poppers) as a stimulant prior to and during sex, which was considered to have a weakening effect on the immune system, and a 'hard-living' approach which involved a combination of an unhealthy diet, drug use and repeated incidences of sexually transmitted disease.

In the end, such assumptions fell down not only because they suggested that all gay men with the condition lived in the same way, which was clearly nonsense, but because AIDS started to affect people who did not identify as gay and whose social and sexual habits bore no resemblance to the 'fast lane' lifestyle upon which the theory rested.

There are, however, those who continue to insist that HIV and AIDS are unrelated. In June 1990, for example, a molecular biologist from the University of California presented the view (on the Channel Four programme *Dispatches*) that the presence of HIV in the bodies of people with AIDS is purely circumstantial. According to Professor Peter Duesberg, HIV is simply an indication of high-risk activities, and is unrelated to the development of AIDS, which occurs only in people whose immune systems have been weakened by unhealthy living. Duesberg backed his claim by saying that viruses work fast (whereas HIV may be in the body for years before - and if - AIDS develops), so that HIV could not therefore be the cause of AIDS.

This view contains obvious flaws, as those angered by the programme's lack of balance were quick to point out. One is that the theory ignores the experience of HIV-positive people in Africa, South America and Asia, where AIDS is unlikely to be related only to malnutrition and persistent infections, since these conditions have existed for a long time whereas AIDS is recognised as a new disorder. Secondly, it is incorrect to say that viruses work fast: there is a mass of evidence to refute this theory - herpes or tuberculosis, for example, lie dormant in the body for years.

But the most obvious problem with arguments that dissociate AIDS from HIV infection is that they fail to address one simple fact. In all people with AIDS HIV is present; people who do not have HIV infection (whatever their lifestyle) do not develop AIDS. Perhaps the most interesting debate to emerge from the *Dispatches* controversy relates less to the validity of Duesberg's ideas than to the responsibility of programme-makers to present a balanced picture of scientists' arguments.

If it is widely recognised that HIV is the cause of AIDS, the origins of the virus remain unclear. It seems likely that it has been around for some years; newspaper reports in 1990 suggested that in 1959 a British sailor died with HIV-related illness.

It is quite possible that we shall never know how or where the virus began. It is also possible that even if we could learn these things the information would not necessarily be of much use to us. What is certain, and what every country in the world now has to face, is that HIV transmission is increasing and will continue to do so until education programmes and control measures such as the screening of blood donations and provision of condoms and clean injecting equipment are able to prevent this.

PATTERNS OF INFECTION

Since 1988, the WHO has chosen to represent the global picture of HIV infection as a combination of three separate patterns of transmission.

1. In North America, Western Europe, Australia and New Zealand, where the vast majority of HIV-positive people were gay men, sex between men was seen as the chief route of spread of the virus (although it was becoming evident that male and female injecting drug users were also showing rising rates of infection). These regions were therefore described as belonging to 'pattern one'.
2. In areas of sub-Saharan Africa, where most people with HIV were heterosexuals considered to be infected through sex, and where transmission from HIV-positive mothers to their children was steadily increasing, 'pattern two' was revealed.
3. 'Pattern three' countries were those where HIV transmission was regarded as relatively limited, occurring mainly as a result of blood transfusion and sexual transmission in the last half of the 1980s, i.e. Eastern Europe, Asia and the Middle East.

The idea of global patterns of this sort was largely a convenience measure to simplify the differing degrees and demographic impact of HIV infection world-wide. However, these patterns are generalised. To begin with, they cannot be viewed as static. Latin America and the Caribbean were initially regarded as pattern one countries, but were later changed by WHO to patterns one *and* two, when the rate of infection among women infected through sex was shown to be growing rapidly. Secondly, it is inappropriate to make assumptions about specific communities as a result of this idea of regional patterns, since HIV infection does not usually affect a population evenly. Thus, although in the majority of African countries HIV is considered to be transmitted primarily through sex between men and women, both the level of infection and the rate of increase of HIV transmission among heterosexuals may vary enormously from one area to another.

WHO statistics, like those collected by the Public Health Laboratory Service in Britain, rely on recorded numbers of people with AIDS to map out general global trends. The difficulty with this is that there is a time lapse of a number of years for any individual between the date of infection with HIV and the point at which he or she may develop illness. Relying on AIDS reports alone inevitably gives an outdated picture of the HIV epidemic. In the absence of detailed and up-to-date statistics for HIV infection world-wide, information about whom HIV is affecting, as well as where and how, remains limited.

There is another sense in which the 'patterns of infection' approach may be less than helpful. It is unlikely that, for example, the idea of HIV transmission rates among gay men will have any global significance, so long as international notions of what sexual orientation implies differ so greatly. The notion of clearly defined distinctions between homosexuality, bisexuality and heterosexuality apparent in epidemiological studies of HIV simply do not apply in many countries. The terms themselves may have little meaning in some regions, where it is acceptable for same-sex relationships to occur but unacceptable for sexual preference to form the basis of any sense of social identity. Even in countries where sexuality has become politicised, and it is possible to speak of a recognisable gay community, men may still have sex with men without regarding themselves as gay, and men who do see themselves as gay may have sex with women. (This of course also applies to lesbians, who as a result of the kind of sexual compartmentalising described above do not feature in the 'patterns of infection' idea, because they are generally regarded to be at very low risk of HIV.)

Presenting the global epidemic in terms of identifiable regional patterns may also become increasingly outdated as HIV becomes more widespread in every area. If we look instead at broad trends of infection internationally, some alarming findings come to light. The most common route of HIV transmission globally is sex between men and women; by 1990 it accounted for about 60 per cent of all cases of HIV infection. By the year 2000, the WHO anticipates that between 75 and 80 per cent of HIV infections will result from unsafe sex between men and women. In the UK alone, the prevalence of HIV among heterosexual men and women almost doubled during 1990.

Women are increasingly at risk, as are young people and infants. According to WHO estimates in November 1990, over 3 million women world-wide are likely to be HIV positive already; AIDS has become the chief cause of death for women aged between 20 and 40 in major cities in the Americas, Western Europe and sub-Saharan Africa. Around 3 million more women may become ill and die with HIV infection during the 1990s.

About one third of reported AIDS cases globally are babies. Since the recorded total of people with AIDS world-wide is likely to be only about half of the actual figure, WHO considers that there could be as many as 400,000 babies whose mothers passed HIV to them during pregnancy, or possibly through breastfeeding. By the year 2000, there may be a cumulative total of 15 to 20 million adults and 10 million infants and children with AIDS world-wide.

The children of adults with HIV face other problems than the risk of infection, however. Even if they remain uninfected themselves, they may well become orphans if their parents die with HIV illness. It is likely that an additional 10 million uninfected children world-wide will be orphaned in this manner during the 1990s. The question of who will care for these children is just one of the unresolved issues raised by the growing impact of the HIV epidemic upon heterosexual adults.

International levels of injecting (and non-injecting) drug use, which are linked especially to the urban areas of both industrialised and developing countries, are also perceived by WHO to be at critical levels. In September 1990, a global programme on drug use was launched by WHO's Director General Dr Hiroshi Nakajima. Nakajima stated that for a large number of countries drug use could represent 'the most serious peace-time threat to well-being in this century . . . by sharing injection needles, millions are being exposed to the threat of infection with the virus that causes AIDS.'

Apart from the direct risk of HIV infection through sharing injecting equipment, the use of drugs may also have an impact on sexual behaviour, since it can induce a sense of indifference towards safer sex practices.

Finally, sexually transmitted diseases (STDs) across the world are considered to have reached epidemic proportions. According to WHO, 250 million or more cases occur each year, constituting a 'public health nightmare'. Around one million of these are new cases of HIV infection, and the increase in STDs generally has two major implications for the spread of HIV. Firstly, if diseases such as gonorrhoea, syphilis, chlamydial infections, genital warts and hepatitis B are more common, it is safe to assume that safer sex is not being widely practised. Secondly, research indicates that the presence of genital lesions caused by STDs may increase the chance of infection with HIV by over 300 per cent.

Such aspects of the epidemic will have an impact on people in every country. Nevertheless, it is the developing world that has been hardest hit by HIV infection. In 1985, about half the people with HIV globally were considered to be from developing countries; by 1990 this figure was nearer two-thirds, and it could reach 75 to 80 per cent by the end of this century. National programmes to control HIV infection and individuals' ability to change their behaviour are affected by questions of economy, politics, religion, culture, and sexual autonomy.

EDUCATION AND INFORMATION

It is possible to make a distinction between *education* and *information* campaigns on HIV and AIDS. Information about HIV may take the form of written materials – leaflets, brochures, posters and so on – as well as publicity directed through mass media such as television, radio, newspapers and billboards. Information campaigns may not involve direct contact with those for whom they are intended, and their frequent aim, i.e. to reach large groups of people quickly, can necessitate simple, general messages that cannot take into account the diversity of social, educational and economic circumstances represented by their audience or readership.

Education campaigns may be seen to involve an interpretative process. They are about providing and clarifying information, but they also aim to examine the *significance* of such information for specific groups; to consider how facts about HIV transmission translate into individual realities. The key messages in education work of this sort are often generated by the very communities at whom they are targetted; alternatively they may be the product of AIDS educators from non-governmental organisations working with local people over sustained periods of time. The emphasis tends to be upon reaching small, culturally-specific groups, building an atmosphere of trust, sharing ideas and skills, and developing an understanding of the factors that may make behaviour change difficult and working to find ways of overcoming these, in on-going projects.

This is not to say that one approach is necessarily preferable to the other, or that they are mutually exclusive: it is possible for community education initiatives to complement mainstream information campaigns. Their goals are different, however. Early research into HIV prevention work suggests that information may raise awareness and change what people *know* about HIV and AIDS; education campaigns are generally considered to have more of an effect on changing what they *do*.

In developing countries, the first attempts to bring HIV and AIDS to the public's attention and to raise levels of knowledge have generally been in the form of government programmes conducted through the mass media. This is likely to be partly due to a lack of resources and training among local communities, which makes them unqualified to take the initiative in HIV prevention work; it is also linked to difficulties in obtaining information.

In contrast, community-based campaigns in industrialised countries have tended to precede national government programmes – for example in the US or UK, where gay men organised themselves to produce relevant literature on staying safe from infection years before there was any sort of public information campaign. And, as opposed to their counterparts in the poorer southern hemisphere, communities existing in the northern hemisphere have often been able to draw upon the advice and expertise of an existing network of voluntary bodies concerned with issues of health, welfare and sexuality.

HIV in the Media

Most governments reporting cases of HIV and AIDS to the World Health Organization have now conducted public information campaigns on the subject, mainly through the mass media. The success of such campaigns depends not just on the messages used or the way in which they are presented, but also on the relationship between the 'target groups' and the medium concerned. As American academic Cindy Patton has pointed out, 'There are highly ritualised ways of interpreting information provided by mass media campaigns.' For example, local radio stations and newspapers in some countries might be seen as giving more 'reliable' information than the national media does, if HIV is perceived to be a specifically local concern.

Economic and political factors may also be involved. In a capitalist economy, mainstream media publicity on HIV may lend the issue extra significance: if the advertisements are known to have cost a lot of money, then the epidemic may be seen as serious enough to merit the expenditure. In countries where press, radio and television are controlled by the government, mass media campaigns may be seen as further evidence of State interference in the lives of individuals - and their messages ignored as a result. In some cases, State-controlled television has said little or nothing about the HIV epidemic. Martin Suchanek, director of a series of Czechoslovakian television advertisements on HIV risks from unsafe sex, said in an interview with the *European* newspaper that 'Before the revolution, the way of life here was very strict and everything was controlled ... we see this campaign as a preventative measure so that our people will realise the risk in this new way of life ... [the AIDS advertisements] certainly would never have been possible when the communists were in power.'

Studies of the different approaches adopted by governments in mass media campaigns suggest that positive messages celebrating the benefits of behaviour change may have a considerably more powerful impact than those relying on scaring people into practising safer sex or safer drug use. A 1990 study by Dr Lorraine Sherr of St Mary's Hospital, London involved showing participants frightening images from a previous Government campaign targetted at drug users, depicting arms being pierced by needles and injecting equipment wrapped in blood-stained gauze. Although the anxiety level of those involved was shown to have increased, the images had no apparent lasting impact on participants' behaviour, perhaps because not one of them was reported to have felt that the advertisements had any personal relevance. Research linked to a 1987 campaign by the Australian Government, involving television advertisements which featured a 'grim reaper' figure of death aiming balls into a bowling alley of human skittles, showed that although the publicity had succeeded in raising levels of awareness of and anxiety about HIV generally it had not prompted safer behaviour.

At a 1988 international summit meeting of Health Ministers, held in London, there was general agreement among delegates that government information campaigns are more likely to be successful if they highlight positive messages rather than negative ones, using humour and an 'upbeat' approach where possible. However, this theory has not necessarily been translated into action. A campaign designed in the late 1980s by the South African Government to warn black people about AIDS featured a poster showing a group of mourners watching a coffin being lowered into the earth, under the slogan 'AIDS - The New Killer Disease is Here.' A poster campaign run by the USSR Health Ministry (women have regularly been blamed for the transmission of HIV and other sexually transmitted diseases in the Soviet Union) presented a collage of fragments of women's bodies - a visual representation of the health threat to men they are seen to represent.

Other attempts by governments to inform the public have been undermined by the use of indirect language and simple lack of information. A French campaign showed posters of teenagers proclaiming that 'Le Sida Ne Passera Pas Par Moi' - or (roughly) 'I'm not going to let it happen to me.' They gave no information about how to stay safe. In Argentina, where media coverage of HIV has been extremely limited, slogans stuck on the side of garbage collection vehicles state that 'La Droga Es Basura' - 'Drugs are Rubbish' - but say nothing about the link between HIV infection and injecting drug use. In the US, the first attempt at a national information campaign - a leaflet called 'America Responds to AIDS' - had to be scrapped in 1987 due to disagreements over appropriate language to educate the public. The American journal *Science* reported that the word 'homosexual' did not appear at all in the leaflet, even though gay men made up 70 per cent of people with AIDS at that time. Other scientists have remarked that the word 'family' appeared far more frequently than the word 'condom'.

In contrast, blunt messages emphasising the possibilities of HIV prevention rather than the dangers of infection appear to have more of an impact. In 1987 the Swiss Government launched its mass media STOP AIDS campaign, where the 'O' of 'STOP' was an image of a rolled-up condom. In January 1990 the campaign extended to advertisements on billboards throughout the country based around the kinds of excuses people make for not using condoms, such as 'They put women off', 'I can't feel anything', 'They destroy the mood', and so on. In each case, the evasive statement was countered with a snappy one-line response. Monitoring of the public's response to these advertisements suggests that awareness of HIV is very high.

Humour may have an important role in dispelling the embarrassment, fear or complacency with which people may view the subject of HIV infection. Television advertisements by the Danish National Board of Health in 1988 highlighted the difficulties some couples may experience in 'negotiating' the use of condoms.

One ad depicted the following: a middle-aged couple are about to have sex, but the woman will not let the man into bed with her until he produces the required rubber. The man's misunderstanding of what she means by 'rubber' leads him to emerge from the bathroom wearing, in turn, a rubber ring, a pair of galoshes, a wetsuit, an inflatable dinghy and finally – in desperation – a condom. Similarly, a cinema advertisement by the British Health Education Authority in late 1990 featured a woman called Mrs Dawson working on a condom production line. She talks about how young people seem to be taking HIV and AIDS messages seriously, as more condoms are being made than ever before – she's never been so busy. At the end, the slogan appears: 'Keep Mrs Dawson busy. Use a condom.'

A few campaigns have chosen to sell safer sex by eroticising the possibilities it presents. A campaign for gay men by the Dutch Government used posters showing attractive photographs of men which emphasised the pleasures of sexual exploration. The Dutch also featured a television advertisement in which a man and a woman in front of a tent, ripping their clothes off in their haste to find the condom, put it on and make love. In Czechoslovakia, a recent campaign by the Department of Health suggests that political changes have been accompanied by a franker approach to sexuality and HIV. In one television advertisement, a naked couple are seen embracing; in another, a male driver is shown picking up a female hitch-hiker. The car disappears behind a hedge. Shortly afterwards the woman's underwear is thrown into the air and viewers see the car rocking up and down.

Reports, features and editorial on HIV and AIDS may be at least as powerful in shaping public awareness as are expensive mass media campaigns, and their role in doing so raises interesting questions about journalistic responsibility and control. In the UK, an insistence by some members of the media on using inaccurate and discriminatory language in HIV/AIDS commentary has led organisations such as the National Union of Journalists and the Non-Governmental Organisations' AIDS Consortium to produce guidelines for HIV and AIDS reporting. Britain is by no means alone in experiencing such problems; on the other hand, not all journalists treat a viral epidemic as a handy vehicle for moralistic speculation and sensationalism. Among the inaccuracies and irresponsibility (some reporters have given the name and personal details of people assumed to be HIV positive, often leading to acute distress and discrimination), there has however also been sensitive, measured coverage.

The differing objectives of AIDS educators and journalists may provide a helpful context in which to examine media misrepresentation. Educators want to focus on simple, basic messages and present them in appealing and appropriate ways so that they 'stick'. The job of journalists is to seek out news, or at least to stimulate interest and excitement (and therefore sales) by providing a new slant on an old subject. They may also be required to present highly technical data in a direct, easy-to-assimilate manner. The problem with reporting HIV/AIDS is that, as far as the basic routes of transmission are concerned, there *is* no new line to take. Routes of transmission have not changed since the epidemic began. The urge to get a good story may, however, be one reason why there has been regular press publicity in the UK and elsewhere about 'casual' transmission through social contact, mosquito bites or even toilet seats.

Similarly, the need for some journalists to simplify complex scientific information has led in some cases to the development of a misleading sort of reporter's 'shorthand', where no distinction is made between HIV infection and AIDS, where the HIV antibody test is described as the 'AIDS test' and where an AIDS diagnosis is portrayed as 'full-blown' or 'frank' AIDS, as if other phases of HIV illness were somehow less significant or even irrelevant.

Commercialism may also play a part. A newspaper has to sell itself, and television or radio programmes need to consider their ratings; they may therefore be concerned with appealing to what are considered mainstream views. Sometimes this has meant allocating blame to people with HIV and AIDS for spreading the virus to others, or the portrayal of illness in terms of innocence and guilt. Chris Gill, editor of the Australian gay community newspaper *The Melbourne Star Observer*, stated in a piece for Canberra's *National AIDS Bulletin* that 'There has been almost no public discussion of what it's actually like to have AIDS, or how it changes an individual's life or of what it's like to have a loved one diagnosed or pass away . . . It is no coincidence that the most honest coverage of AIDS . . . has been in the non-commercial media.'

Sometimes radio and television entertainment play an informal but important role in generating awareness. An television soap opera in the Phillipines featuring the relationship between a businessman with HIV and his partner resulted in a 100 per cent rise in the numbers of people attending STD clinics in Manila the week after the relevant episode was broadcast. During 1990 and 1991, the British soap opera *Eastenders* ran a continuing storyline about a central character, Mark Fowler, finding out that he was HIV positive and being afraid to tell his family. For the first few weeks of the story, the Terrence Higgins Trust received around three times as many information requests from the public as usual.

Ultimately, journalists are members of the public, who may sympathise with the prejudices and ignorance of public opinion. They need not agree that they have a responsibility to change ideas and shape behaviour with respect to HIV infection and the people who live with it. In this they are considerably at odds with the view of many health professionals. Dr Edward Naganu, permanent secretary in Botswana's Health Ministry, told delegates at an 'AIDS and Media' workshop that his inclination was to blame the mass media for misinformation: 'I could say they like sensationalism, they exaggerate, they want privileged information and they enjoy embarrassing people. I don't know if these allegations are true. But this is definitely the perception of many health workers.'

Education in the Community

In contrast to large-scale public information campaigns, education initiatives provided by local people and organisations are often able to engage interest and motivate behaviour change in areas where HIV prevention messages might otherwise have little impact. A high level of illiteracy and lack of access to television and radio are often factors that limit the success of mass media advertising and printed materials in raising awareness about HIV and AIDS. Community education projects in both developing and industrialised countries have tended to involve multiple channels of communication; they may use songs, theatre, dance, puppetry and games to present their points of view.

In less developed nations these initiatives frequently operate at a grassroots level, involving people who are well-respected within the community - tribal leaders, midwives, members of the church and so on. The people for whom the project is intended participate, discussing their information needs, the problems they may face in making sexual activity or drug use safer, and the appropriate language, images and media necessary to get ideas across to others. Since financial resources for such projects are often scarce, they may have to be extremely cheap to run, or even cost-free.

Increasingly, education projects world-wide are built upon a 'peer education' approach. In other words, those involved are provided with the support, information and training necessary to become effective educators for other people with a common background and level of understanding of HIV/AIDS within their community. In the process, all participants gain confidence and skills which may make personal behaviour change a little easier. In Thailand, which has around 500,000 female prostitutes, HIV infection is rapidly on the increase. Local sex-worker groups such as *Empower* in Bangkok have organised safer sex cabarets and condom-inflating competitions in Patpong bars for prostitutes and their clients. There are similar projects in places as far apart as Nairobi and Birmingham, where women with a background in the sex industry share condoms and literature about safer sex and drug use, as well as their own advice and experience. In Zambia, anti-AIDS clubs in schools have given students a chance to inform each other, a model of education which has now been adopted in other African countries.

Experience has shown repeatedly that people with HIV often make the most effective educators. Their ability to lend credibility and force to educational campaigns derives not just from direct experience of HIV infection but from an understanding of how to approach and inform their own communities. Richard Rector, an American living with AIDS who now works for the Norwegian Red Cross, said at an international AIDS information conference in 1989 that people with HIV and AIDS can play a vital role in breaking down boundaries between people, generating greater understanding about dangerous attitudes and behaviours, and working towards a safer, less discriminatory future for people with the virus as well as those at risk of infection. According to Rector, HIV illness has been seen as 'other people's disease – it's time to bring the message home to those who see it as "out there", nothing to do with them.'

In San Francisco, an education programme called 'The Wedge' brings people with AIDS into schools to talk to students about the condition. In Kenya, an organisation run by Robert Mugemana, a man with AIDS, provides counselling, support and information to anybody who needs it, in an attempt to give AIDS what Mugemana calls 'a human face and a form' to which people can relate.

Community education initiatives may be constrained by a weak economy, especially in developing countries. There may be a chronic shortage of clean needles and syringes, HIV antibody testing kits and condoms. For people with HIV illness, drug treatments, hospital care, counselling and support may be severely limited, and sometimes non-existent. Thus the most powerful campaigns to raise awareness about safer behaviour can fail. So may those which aim to prevent stigmatisation of people with HIV: when economic factors undermine an individual's ability to stay safe, prejudice and hostility towards those who are HIV positive become easier.

In Uganda, where posters, brochures and radio carry the message 'Love Carefully' (a slogan that has now become famous internationally), the AIDS Control Programme estimates that around 1.2 million people are HIV positive. It is thought that around 10 million condoms have been imported and made available through family planning clinics and some chemists in the past five years; however, this is hopelessly few in a country where doctors estimate that up to 2 million acts of sexual intercourse take place every day. In the USSR, an AIDS education bulletin called *SPID-Info* (SPID means AIDS in the Soviet Union) ran a comic strip in late 1990 comparing the national 'condom situation' with that in the US. It was based around a 'boy-meets-girl' situation. In the American story, the boy rushes off to buy condoms when it becomes clear he will need them. In the Soviet story, the boy does the round of every pharmacy he can find, but no condoms are available. The story ends with the boy committing suicide in a state of frustration.

An over-burdened economy, often resulting in acute poverty among some social groups, may take its toll in other ways. In many countries, young children are forced onto the streets as a result of the death of their parents, the threat of sexual abuse or other factors. They may find that selling sex is the only way to survive; some may also get involved in drug use. Such children are often particularly difficult to reach with education and support programmes because they do not go to school and may be suspicious of the approaches of adults. The Survivors' Project, a Canadian-based scheme which works with street children internationally, has created films and cartoons about staying safe from HIV infection using the ideas and perspectives that emerge from spending time with the children in their own environment. Peter Dalglish, a co-ordinator of the project, says that the language and content of such materials is unashamedly explicit. They were made for the poorest children in the world, and for them sexual exploitation, drug use and rape are the harsh realities of day-to-day life.

Political oppression often goes hand-in-hand with economic hardship, and can further undermine attempts to halt the spread of HIV. The struggle for democracy in Eastern Europe has brought to light the legacies of restrictive health and social policies and government denial of HIV and AIDS. In Romania, which by April 1991 reported 1,226 people with AIDS to the WHO – by far the highest number recorded in Eastern Europe – the policy of the late President Ceausescu that abortion and contraception should be banned so that families could produce at least five children each resulted in over 100,000 children being dumped in state orphanages by parents who could not afford or did not want to have them. Many of the children were suffering from illness and nutritional problems, and were given blood transfusions to boost their health. Tragically, it had the opposite effect: contaminated blood supplies and unsterilised injecting equipment were used, so that around 1,000 of these children became infected with HIV.

Religion exerts a strong influence on HIV education projects world-wide, for better and for worse. The Church is integral to the lives of millions of people, and may have networks that allow information to reach remote areas where state-run institutions have no effect. Churches also have credibility and power, especially in Latin America and Africa. In Uganda, about 92 per cent of the population are thought to be actively involved with one Church or another. The traditional role of the Church in caring for sick and dying people has played an important part in countries such as Zambia, where HIV information leaflets like 'Choose to Live' emphasise the fact that social contact cannot transmit the virus, and state the need 'not to isolate (people with HIV) but to give them better medical, moral and spiritual support'.

However, religious doctrine may often undermine rather than facilitate the efforts of HIV educators. Despite figures released by the WHO revealing that at least 5 million people in Africa are already infected with HIV, while on a tour of four African countries in September 1990 the Pope announced his opposition to the use of condoms for HIV prevention, stating that they would only encourage 'the very behaviour which has greatly contributed to the expansion of the disease'. In Spain, where a £3-million Government campaign uses the snappily-named 'Semen Up' pop group to promote the message 'Pontelo – Ponselo' – 'Put one on – Put one on him', the Church and family organisations have accused the Government of 'promoting the sexual act' and trying to take teenagers away from parental control.

Islamic fundamentalism in parts of Africa and the Arab Middle East has often led to AIDS prevention work receiving a low priority in order to avoid offending the sensibilities of Muslim society. According to Islamic beliefs, extra-marital sex, prostitution and homosexuality are unacceptable, while condoms may be used only for family planning purposes. Thus HIV prevention campaigns avoid any discussion of safer sex; they focus instead on chastity, and fidelity within marriage.

Cultural attitudes (which are often shaped by religious beliefs) are of tremendous importance in determining the success of HIV education initiatives. To an increasingly important degree, the sexual and social status afforded to women throughout the world is shaping the course of the HIV epidemic. Women are often the key providers of health care within their families and local communities, yet their own health and welfare needs may be seen as of secondary importance. Research from the US suggests that women with HIV are diagnosed later and survive for shorter periods of time than do men with the virus; the disparity is attributed to an imbalance in access to health care and inadequate understanding of women's symptoms of infection, rather than biological differences between the sexes.

At the same time, women's ability to protect their health is constrained by limited access to education. In many developing countries priority is given to educating men, so illiteracy levels among women may remain high. There is also the question of women's sexual autonomy. According to Ernesto de la Vega of the Brooklyn AIDS Task Force, Puerto Rican women, as others, may be afraid to discuss sex with their male partners, on whom they may also be financially dependent. Women fear violence or rejection; they may be afraid that raising the question of condoms will lead to accusations that they have been unfaithful, or that they consider their partner to be unfaithful. In any case, limited sex education may leave many women with scant awareness of the sexual choices open to them, and a sense that it is improper to make demands upon their partner. 'For some of the poorest Latina women, sex is something which happens to them in the dark and in silence,' says de la Vega.

The most successful educational approaches are those which have challenged the cultural assumptions that limit women's lives. The Victoria Prostitute's Collective in Australia runs a 'Hello sailor' campaign providing HIV education for servicemen. Cheryl Overs of the Collective fiercely contests the view that women selling sex should be seen as a 'reservoir' of HIV infection for their clients. She feels that 'Safer sex is the only option for women sex workers like everyone else . . . the fact that money changes hands is neither here nor there. The virus doesn't travel on dollar bills.' A sex education booklet published by the Native American Women's Health Centre in South Dakota stresses self-esteem and assertiveness skills. It shows a man and a woman in conversation. 'I can make you feel like a real woman,' says the man. 'No,' she responds, 'I'm already a woman without your help.'

Above all, HIV prevention projects are likely to be of little value unless they acknowledge the circumstances that have an impact on sexual and drug-using behaviour. For men and women whose lives are curtailed by factors such as homelessness or acute poverty, the need for safer behaviour may seem of limited importance. As Marie St Cyr, a counsellor working with drug-using men and women in New York City has said: 'If the only ways of escape people have are through drugs and sex . . . and both of these are very closely linked with AIDS, then what hope is there of addressing AIDS prevention without addressing the underlying issue of what people are trying to escape from?'

HIV AND HUMAN RIGHTS

Epidemics have always played a powerful role in shaping health and social policy. They may lead to a stronger collaboration between health organisations, local and national government; they may prompt important advances in health care such as the development of vaccination programmes. They may also involve the enforcement of coercive measures, as with the imposition of enforced isolation for people with cholera during the nineteenth century.

With regard to the HIV epidemic, it is evident that the provision of information on its own is unlikely to be adequate to slow the spread of infection. As discussed in this chapter, behaviour change is determined by factors more complex than the availability of educational materials, and can often be a slow and difficult process. While many people would agree that education programmes are most effective when supported by relevant public health measures (such as screening of blood donations, provision of condoms and clean injecting equipment and voluntary testing programmes), governments all over the world have been prompted to seek a solution to HIV transmission in policies which severely undermine the rights of people living with the virus.

The Panos Institute, an international information and policy studies organisation, makes an important distinction between 'inclusive' and 'exclusive' approaches to HIV prevention. 'Exclusive' approaches are identified as those which prevent people with HIV from enjoying the same degree of freedom as do other members of society, in order to protect the health of those who are uninfected. 'Inclusive' approaches are based on the principle that there is an important connection between slowing the spread of HIV and the protection of the rights of all individuals: thus the experience, knowledge and insight of people with HIV is seen as one of the most powerful and valuable resources available in HIV prevention policy.

There is no strong evidence from anywhere in the world that policies such as the compulsory testing of groups seen to be 'high risk', the imposition of immigration restrictions on people with HIV, or the enforced separation of those who have tested HIV positive from those deemed to be uninfected have been of any benefit in preventing further cases of infection. Yet the restrictions continue.

Compulsory Testing is discussed briefly in Chapter 6 of this book. In some cases it may be imposed upon specific groups, in others it may be enforced more widely. While countries such as Guatemala, Israel and Austria (among others) now test prostitute women for HIV infection, the Cuban Government is currently embarking on a programme to test its entire population. Those found to be HIV positive are placed in isolation from friends, partners and families, in special sanitoria 'until there's a cure'. Bulgaria too, has proposed a mass testing programme for all its citizens, but this has been postponed temporarily due to a shortage of testing kits. In the US, a large number of states compel people convicted of prostitution, or of selling or using drugs illegally, to take the HIV antibody test. There are further examples of such programmes, from most regions of the world, too numerous to mention here.

In many ways, compulsory testing raises more questions than it answers. There is, for example, the question of personal responsibility. It can be argued that since information about HIV transmission routes is now fairly widespread, an individual who is HIV negative has as much responsibility to stay uninfected as a person with HIV has not to pass the virus on. Also, as discussed in Chapter 6, compulsory testing programmes are inefficient as a means of HIV surveillance because the 'window of infection' period between the date of infection and development of HIV antibodies will always render inaccurate a proportion of the test results. Since the HIV antibody test is never 100 per cent accurate in any case, large scale compulsory testing programmes would produce a substantial number of false positive results.

Testing programmes are also expensive, particularly when balanced against the numbers of people with HIV they may reveal. In the US, a pre-marital HIV testing programme for couples in

Illinois was calculated to have cost around US $208,000 for each identified case of HIV infection. It is also considered to have resulted in a large number of men and women simply applying to get married in other states, in order to avoid the need for a test. In some countries, the question of wide-scale testing programmes does not arise: there is barely the money to provide tests for those who want them, let alone those who may not.

Another example of the attempt to control HIV transmission by social division is the introduction of certificates or cards stating an individual's HIV antibody status. Private health clinics in the UK, which provide the test in return for a fee – counselling generally costs extra – have offered an 'AIDS-free' card as part of their service. Similarly, sex workers in Bangkok, Thailand, may be tested and issued with cards stamped in blue or red. If a woman's stamp is blue, this implies that it is all right for clients to have unprotected sex with her.

As with compulsory testing, this approach to prevention ignores the fact that test results may be inaccurate, for reasons described above. It ignores the range of possibilities offered by safer sex, suggesting instead that people with HIV should not have sexual relationships at all. In any case, certification of this sort could never be up to date: a person with an 'AIDS-free' card today might become HIV positive tomorrow.

Selective isolation and *mass isolation* of people with HIV involve, respectively, detaining people who know that they are HIV positive but continue to practise unsafe behaviour, and universal isolation of all people with HIV infection (as in the Cuban sanitoria) from those who are HIV negative. Selective isolation tends to operate on a temporary basis: in Sweden, a female sex worker has been sentenced to isolation several times because she continues to work in the red light areas of Stockholm even though she has been prohibited from doing so by the administrative court. She was sentenced despite her insistence that she only provides safer sex and always uses condoms. In India, there are similar examples. A detention centre in Madras continues to hold women prostitutes with HIV, many of whom have little awareness of what their infection means and less idea of when they will be released. Some have been held for up to six years.

It can be argued that selective isolation is justifiable if voluntary measures fail, because governments have a public duty to protect people against transmission of disease. However, it is certainly not without problems. It may not always be possible to judge, for example, whether a person with HIV knew of his or her infection before the 'unsafe behaviour' occurred; as with the case of the Swedish prostitute, whether or not a person has behaved unsafely is also open to interpretation. Again, the question of responsibility in sexual relationships arises: does it lie solely with the person with HIV, or is it to be shared? There is scope for abuse in such cases – if a person is deemed to be dangerous to others, he or she may be held in isolation on the grounds of what *might* happen in the future, rather than as the result of current behaviour.

The imposition of restrictions on international travel for people with HIV has become increasingly common, although a resolution passed by the World Health Assembly (the governing body of the World Health Organization) in May 1988 called upon member states to avoid this and other kinds of discrimination. Such restrictions generally take the form of requiring foreign nationals to provide evidence of being HIV negative before they are granted entry to a country; sometimes this also applies to citizens returning from abroad.

There are a number of reasons why such travel restrictions are ineffective in preventing transmission of HIV. As a WHO consultation paper on the subject has stated, the enormous number of people who now travel internationally makes a system of applying tests to travellers 'extraordinarily complex and prone to error of many sorts, including false exclusion of uninfected individuals and a false "clean bill of health" for some HIV-infected persons'. Furthermore, WHO points out that the need for counselling about behaviour change and confidentiality regarding HIV status (which must be regarded as important ethical considerations) would be impossible to meet on such a vast scale. As with 'HIV-free' certification discussed above, a passport stamped with an entry visa has no impact upon an individual's behaviour once he or she has arrived in a country.

It is extremely likely that coercion will not prove to be a useful HIV prevention tool, quite apart from the distress it may generate. Testing and isolation of specific groups, for example, may lead others not identified as 'high risk' to disregard the possibility of infection, and therefore to make no effort to practise safer behaviour. At the same time, if people who see themselves as at risk of HIV (or who already have symptoms of illness) are afraid to approach relevant services for advice and support, opportunities to promote health education messages will be wasted, and many people with HIV illness may go uncared for and untreated.

Action to Protect Human Rights

Since the HIV epidemic began, the rights of HIV-positive people have been a major focus of attention. Activist groups (based mainly in the US and Western Europe) have become increasingly articulate and effective in improving the welfare of people with HIV by campaigning for quicker, fairer and more widely available drug treatment trials, adequate housing and health care, and so on.

At the 6th Global Conference on AIDS, held in San Francisco, 15 British voluntary organisations called for the rights of people with HIV infection to be protected by an international convention. Jonathan Grimshaw, Director of the London's Landmark Centre for people with HIV and author of the declaration, stated that all the rights listed in the document were already spelled out in international treaties to which Britain is a subscriber. These include the right to privacy, liberty and security, freedom of movement, equal protection under the law and protection from discrimination, the right to employment, housing, food, education, medical help and welfare, and the right to marry. A further clause called for the free access of people with HIV and AIDS to a 'database providing information about therapeutic research' and 'access to medical treatments and drugs'.

There has been increasing interest in the potential of international human rights law to safeguard the rights of people with HIV and AIDS. In 1989, the United Nations Centre for Human Rights and WHO's Global Program on AIDS organised an International Consultation to discuss AIDS and human rights. Its Final Document concluded that interference with the right to liberty, security, privacy and freedom of movement are inconsistent with international human rights standards. Measures such as voluntary HIV antibody testing, pre- and post-test counselling of individuals, voluntary drug treatment programmes for HIV infection and voluntary changes in behaviour among HIV-positive people could, on the other hand, be regarded as consistent with such standards.

One of the difficulties with the international application of human rights is that there is no single court with jurisdiction over the world's sovereign states, nor any means to enforce the judgement of such a court if it existed. Nevertheless, there is certainly scope for international human rights law to be of use to people with HIV infection. The fact that the vast majority of people with HIV are unaware of the protection of their rights offered by such law should be a key challenge for future HIV education programmes.

QUESTIONS OF RESPONSIBILITY

The history of the HIV epidemic presents us with so many unanswered questions. As Dr Anthony Fauci, director of the US National Institute of Allergy and Infectious Diseases, has stated, 'If the 1980s was the decade of AIDS, I can assure you that 1990s will be the second decade of AIDS.' The epidemic is not going to dwindle in the foreseeable future; the questions will remain.

Some of these questions relate to the availability of drug treatments for people with HIV infection and illness: Why are women and black people under-represented among participants in drug treatment trials? What can be done to help people with HIV in countries which cannot afford to provide such drugs at all? How long will it be before scientists can produce a treatment which will be entirely safe and effective in preventing illness in people with HIV infection?

Other questions refer to education and research programmes: How can people be persuaded to make changes in their behaviour if they are not helped to overcome the circumstances that may make such changes difficult or even impossible? If funding for HIV research is limited, what balance should be struck between financing scientific studies and financing further analyses of the factors that influence attitudes and awareness? Will HIV education programmes for young people be able to present sexual relationships in an honest and positive light, so that safer sex is seen as a source of excitement and potential rather than restriction?

Still other questions concern economics: What and how much should the richer countries of the world do to support those whose under-resourced health services may help to increase the spread of HIV infection? How will poorer nations cope in the future with the costs of care for people with HIV illness? As the epidemic continues internationally, will the financial burden of health service provision mean that care for HIV-positive people will become a matter of personal wealth rather than individual need?

These are questions of individual and collective responsibility. In the same way that the view that the rights of a minority – those with HIV infection – must be jeopardised in order to protect the rights of an uninfected majority is a false premise upon which to base HIV prevention policy, so is the notion that the health of the world's people can be anything other than a global concern. The future of the HIV epidemic will be determined by the degree and willingness with which individuals and governments can share information, acknowledge mistakes, and work together for change.

DIRECTORY OF FURTHER READING AND RESOURCES

PUBLICATIONS – BOOKS

The following list is in no way comprehensive; there is an enormous amount of literature available on HIV and AIDS. Newsletters in particular are numerous, and it may be worthwhile to contact a local HIV agency to find out what is available in your area. The titles mentioned here should provide interesting and helpful further reading.

General

The AIDS Handbook – Carl Miller, London: Penguin, 1990. By the country's first AIDS liaison officer, this is an excellent general guide to HIV issues.

The Search for the Virus: the Scientific Discovery of AIDS and the Quest for a Cure – Steve Connor and Sharon Kingman, London: Penguin, 1988 (revised 1989). A highly readable and interesting account of the social and biomedical issues relating to HIV. Connor and Kingman were previously AIDS reporters for the *New Scientist*.

Living with HIV Infection

AIDS: A Guide to Survival – Peter Tatchell, London: Gay Men's Press, 1990. Good exploration of practical ways of staying healthy with HIV infection; particularly strong on alternative therapies.

Living with AIDS – Stephen R. Graubard (ed.), Cambridge, MA: MIT Press, 1990. A meaty and extremely wide-ranging set of essays on medical, social and political aspects of HIV infection in the US, this is no lightweight read, but well worth the effort.

Living with AIDS and HIV – David Miller, Basingstoke: Macmillan, 1987. One of those simply written and practical books about dealing with the medical and psychological impact of HIV that continues to be relevant and interesting.

Caring

Caring for Someone with AIDS – Research Institute for Consumer Affairs/Disabilities Study Unit, London: Hodder and Stoughton, 1990. Probably the most comprehensive and sensible guide to care issues so far, this is an indispensable resource both for the person living with HIV and the carer.

AIDS: A Strategy for Nursing Care - Robert Pratt, London: Edward Arnold Ltd, 1988. Strong summary of biomedical information, and useful information on treatment drugs. Takes patient-centred approach.

Women

Safer Sex - the Guide for Women Today - Diane Richardson, London: Pandora, 1990. Although not just about HIV, there is a useful section on the subject, and much other helpful information besides.

Women and the AIDS Crisis - Diane Richardson, London: Pandora, 1989. This is a new edition of a book first published in 1987. Still the most comprehensive UK book to look at women and HIV.

Triple Jeopardy: Women and AIDS - Panos Institute, London: Panos Publications, 1990. A sharply written and thought-provoking book about the three key ways in which HIV may threaten women, and the implications of this for women internationally.

Women, AIDS and Activism - ACT UP New York Women and AIDS Book Group, Boston, MA: South End Press, 1990. A unique collection of pieces by women activists covering the medical, social and economic aspects of women's experience of the HIV epidemic. There is no British equivalent. Fascinating and powerful.

Drug Use

Facing Up to AIDS - John Mordaunt, Dublin: O'Brien Press, 1989. Mordaunt's account of his past as an injecting drug user, and current AIDS diagnosis. A forceful memoir.

AIDS, Drugs and Prostitution - Martin A. Plant (ed.), London: Tavistock/Routledge, 1990. A set of studies involving sex workers and injecting drug users, this draws some important conclusions about HIV transmission and health policy.

Children

The Impact of AIDS - Ewan Armstrong, London: Gloucester Press, 1989. A book for children.

The Implications of AIDS for Children in Care - Daphne Batty (ed.), London: British Agencies for Adoption and Fostering, 1987. An excellent review, this book remains useful.

Caring for Children with HIV and AIDS - Rosie Claxton and Tony Harrison (eds.), London: Edward Arnold.

International

The Third Epidemic: Repercussions of the Fear of AIDS - Panos Institute, London: Panos Publications, 1990. Comprehensive and extremely interesting presentation of the general impact of HIV upon human rights, as well as detailed information about how each region of the world has responded to the epidemic.

AIDS and the Third World - Panos Institute, London: Panos Publications, 1988. A helpful guide to how developing countries have been affected by HIV. Statistics and other details may be out-of-date now, but it gives a good general picture.

Sex and Sexuality

Safer Sex: A New Look at Sexual Pleasure - Peter Gordon and Louise Mitchell, London: Faber & Faber, 1988. A straightforward, lively and extremely useful discussion of all aspects of sexual pleasure.

Political

Taking Liberties - Erica Carter and Simon Watney (eds.), London: Serpent's Tail Press, 1989. A collection of essays covering the political and social dimension of the HIV epidemic in the UK and US.

Policing Desire: Pornography, AIDS and the Media - Simon Watney, London: Methuen, 1987. An impassioned and highly critical study of the way in which the British and American media have interpreted HIV, and an exploration of the impact of the HIV epidemic and the 'meanings' forced on to it upon the sexuality of gay men.

AIDS and the Good Society - Patricia Illingsworth, London: Routledge, 1990. A philosophical analysis of personal morality and other social issues connected with HIV.

AIDS and Its Metaphors - Susan Sontag, London: Allen Lane, 1989. Brilliant and concise discussion of the misleading imagery that has shaped beliefs about HIV.

Sex and Germs - Cindy Patton, Boston, MA: South End Press, 1985. Patton's presentation of the social and political questions raised by the HIV epidemic is an exciting and challenging read.

The National AIDS Manual - Peter Scott et al., NAM Publications, PO Box 99, London SW2 - is the most comprehensive reference resource available to anyone working in the field of HIV. It comes in two volumes and is enormously detailed, combining hard information on all aspects of HIV infection with a thorough list of organisations and other resources available in the UK and internationally. It is, however, not cheap at £195 for new subscribers (£55 for voluntary organisations), although there are two annual updates. State-of-the-art HIV information.

PUBLICATIONS - NEWSLETTERS

The AIDS Newsletter - Bureau of Hygiene and Tropical Diseases. A fortnightly collection of summarised reports from a wide range of publications, covering UK and international news, prevention measures, health education, and scientific developments including day treatment news. There is also editorial on key items of interest. Highly useful.

HIV News Review - Terrence Higgins Trust. A quarterly newspaper providing an update of all aspects of HIV infection, including reviews of new resources, comment and features.

Body Positive Newsletter - Body Positive. A valuable resource offering information on a range of issues for people living with HIV, as well as details of new services. Strong on treatment issues.

World AIDS - Panos Institute. Excellent bi-monthly giving the latest news, statistics and a detailed report also. The best international news magazine on HIV available in the UK.

Please note: many useful publications on HIV and AIDS are available on a reference basis from the Terrence Higgins Trust library (see p. 247).

SERVICES

For reasons of shortage of space, this is nowhere near a full list of the organisations available throughout the UK. It has been necessary to limit the list to some of the key national organisations working in the field of HIV infection and to agencies not specifically linked to HIV but whose services are nevertheless relevant. For full details of local and national services, contact the Terrence Higgins Trust. Services are listed in alphabetical order.

ACT UP

Activist organisation set up at the end of 1988 to promote human rights for people living with HIV through civil protest and direct action.

ACT UP London – Meetings every Tuesday at the London Lesbian and Gay Centre, 69 Cowcross St, London EC1

Write:
BM Box 2995, London WC1N 3XX
Phone:
071 490 5749

AIDS Ahead

National self-help umbrella group for over 15 different organisations for deaf people. Services include provision of information to deaf people on all aspects of HIV and AIDS; advisory, befriending and support services; grants; training; interpreting services; publications and videos for deaf people.

Write:
144 London Road, Northwich, Cheshire CW9 5HH
Phone:
0606 47047 (direct line)
0606 47831 (Voice or Minicom, plus answerphone)

AIDS and Housing Project

Service to all agencies working in public or voluntary housing in the UK. Provides consultancy, training, production of backup materials, and policies/codes of practice on all matters relating to housing people with HIV.

Write:
AIDS and Housing Project, 16–18 Strutton Ground, London SW1P 2HP
Phone:
071 222 6932, Monday to Friday, 10 a.m. to 6 p.m.

AVERT – AIDS Education and Research Trust

AVERT is a charity aiming to prevent people becoming HIV positive, and improve the quality of life for people who have HIV infection. Services include provision of health education leaflets, as well as funds for educational and research projects.

Write:
PO Box 91, Horsham, West Sussex, RH13 7YR
Phone:
0403 864010, Monday to Friday 9 a.m. to 5 p.m.

Immunity

A charity providing a legal resource and advice centre for people with (or suspected of having) HIV. Offers advice, home and hospital visits, research, and educational materials.

Write:
260a Kilburn Lane, London W10 4BA
Phone:
081 968 8909

Lantern Trust

Charity launched in 1989 to provide training on HIV/AIDS for professional carers. It runs a range of courses, including in-house training, and provides educational materials.

Write:
72 Honey Lane, Waltham Abbey, Essex EN9 3BS
Phone:
0992 714900

Mainliners

Agency for anyone affected by HIV and drugs (including alcohol); promotes self-help approach. Services include education and training; advice; helpline; consultancy; counselling; newsletter; support group; leaflets and posters.

Write:
Mainliners Ltd, PO Box 125, London SW9 8EF
Phone:
071 274 4000, ext. 443

Names Project UK

The British branch of the US Names Project, which produces a quilt made from panels commemorating the lives and names of people with HIV who have died. Will provide information about the project and how to contribute panels.

Write:
797 Christchurch Road, Boscombe, Bournemouth, Dorset BH7 6AW (Send sae)
Phone:
0202 432005 (daytime)
0202 433190 (evenings)

National AIDS Helpline

Twenty-four hour free phoneline offering information and referrals on any aspect of HIV/AIDS. All enquiries answered, and research undertaken if they cannot answer your question. Minicom facilities available, also community information in Asian sub-continent languages, Chinese and Arabic.

Phone:
0800 282 446 (Chinese (Cantonese) and English), Tuesdays 6 p.m. to 10 p.m.
0800 282 445 (Bengali, Hindi, Punjabi, Urdu and English), Wednesdays 6 p.m. to 10 p.m.

0800 282 447 (Arabic and English), Wednesdays 6 p.m. to 10 p.m.

National AIDS Trust

Launched in 1987, NAT's aims are to promote and co-ordinate education initiatives on a wide range of issues. It provides funds for voluntary groups, advises organisations, and acts as link between voluntary and statutory organisations. Produces *AIDS Matters*, a quarterly newsletter.

Write:
14th Floor, Euston Tower, 286 Euston Road, London NW1 3DN
Phone:
071 383 4246

National HIV Prevention Information Service

Information service launched in Spring 1990 to service specialist information needs of health service, local authority and voluntary sector HIV prevention workers.

Write:
82–86 Seymour Place, London W1H 5DB
Phone:
071 724 7993

Scottish AIDS Monitor (SAM)

This was set up in 1983, and is a national HIV charity for the whole of Scotland. Services include buddying and practical help for people with HIV (buddying also covers people in prison); face-to-face counselling; welfare rights and legal advice; health education and training; support groups; speakers; leaflets; safer sex roadshow; newsletter.

Write:
SAM National Office, PO Box 48, Edinburgh EH1 3SA
Phone:
031 557 3885

Terrence Higgins Trust

The first national voluntary organisation providing services on HIV and AIDS. Services provided include buddying; helper cells; face-to-face counselling; legal and welfare rights advice; special fund for people with HIV illness; prison visiting; library and information services (including two newsletters); speakers; hospitality network for people visiting relatives and partners in hospital; support groups; health education initiatives.

Write:
52–54 Gray's Inn Road, London WC1X 8JU
Phone:
071 831 0330

Groups for People with HIV

Body Positive

The first group run for people who are HIV antibody positive. Services include telephone helpline; newsletter; hospital visiting; drop-in centre offering a range of advice and information (legal, social services benefits, health, welfare rights); library; massage; therapy groups; small grants fund; special support groups; speakers; transport.

Phone:
071 835 1045
Drop-in centre:
51b Philbeach Gardens, Earls Court, London SW5 9EB. Times: Monday and Friday - 11 a.m. to 9 p.m.; Tuesday to Thursday - 11 a.m. to 5 p.m.; Sunday - noon to 5 p.m.

Positively Women

The first organisation for HIV-positive women nationally. Provides support groups (including one for Afro-Caribbean women); telephone and face-to-face counselling; buddying; consultancy on service development; education leaflets; children's fund for children of mothers with HIV who have financial problems.

Write:
5 Sebastian St, London EC1V 0HE
Phone:
071 490 1690

HIV Care Centres and Hospices

Landmark

A walk-in centre for people with HIV/AIDS in south London, especially Southwark, Lewisham and Wandsworth. A social centre that aims to develop an extremely flexible service tailored to the needs of the local communities.

Write:
57a Tulse Hill, London SW2
Phone:
081 678 6686

London Lighthouse

A major support and residential centre for people with AIDS which provides an integrated range of services. These include a drop-in area, garden and café; support groups; creative and complementary therapy groups; day-care; training; home support service; housing; residential unit; information service; legal advice; welfare advice; newsletter and many others.

Write:
111-117 Lancaster Road, London W11 1QT
Phone:
071 792 1200

Mildmay Mission Hospital

A Christian charitable hospital caring for young disabled people and adults and children with HIV illness. There is a hospice unit, home and day-care services, as well as educational courses.

Write:
Hackney Road, London E2 7NA
Phone:
071 739 2331

Ethnic/Language-specific Organisations

Black HIV and AIDS Network (BHAN)

The only national organisation providing HIV services for Asian, African and Afro-Caribbean people. These include support groups; home and community care; multilingual counselling; education and training courses; policy development work; seminars and conferences.

Write:
111 Devonport Road, London W12 8PB
Phone:
081 742 9223/081 749 2828

Blackliners Helpline

Support and counselling service for people affected by HIV from Africa, the Caribbean, and Asia, who are living in Britain. Helpline; face-to-face counselling; leaflets and posters; practical help and support to people with HIV; self-help discussion and support groups planned.

Write:
PO Box 1274, London SW9 8EZ
Phone:
071 738 5274 (Helpline), Monday to Friday 9.30 a.m. to 4 p.m. (plus answerphone)

Agencies for Sex Workers

CLASH – Central London Action on Street Health

Project working in all areas of health, including HIV and AIDS. CLASH works with people who might find it difficult to get good health care, such as drug users, sex workers, homeless people and so on. Offers advice, counselling, training and referrals. Can offer condoms and emergency packs of needles.

Write:
CLASH, 15 Batemans Buildings, Soho Hospital, Soho Square, London W1V 5TW
Phone:
071 734 1794, Monday to Friday 10 a.m. to 4.30 p.m., plus answerphone

Streetwise

Charity counselling and helping young men (16 to 21 years old) who sell sex. Provides day centre for those under 21, offers laundry, refreshments, midday meals, weekly doctor's surgery and education and safer sex and drug use.

Write:
Flat 3B, Langham Mansions, Earls Court Square, London SW5 9UP
Phone:
071 373 8860 (Helpline), Monday to Friday 10 a.m. to 5 p.m.
071 370 0406 (Centre) Monday to Friday 11 a.m. to 5 p.m.

Counselling and Support

British Association for Counselling

Publishes a directory of national and local counselling agencies and directory of training available to counselling agencies.

Write:
BAC, 37a Sheep Street, Rugby, Warwickshire, CV21 3BX
Phone:
0788 578328/578329 (Monday to Friday)

Childline

Freefone number for young people in trouble or danger. Support, advice and counselling provided.

Write:
Freepost 1111, London N1 OBR (no stamp needed)
Phone:
0800 1111

Cruse

National organisation offering bereavement counselling, information and support to anyone who needs it.

Write:
Cruse House, 126 Sheen Road, Richmond, Surrey TW9 1UR
Phone:
081 940 4818 (Monday to Friday 9.30 a.m. to 5 p.m.)

Gay Bereavement Project

Telephone support, advice and counselling to lesbians and gay men experiencing bereavement, by lesbians and gay men.

Phone:
081 455 8894 (7 p.m. to midnight every night)

Rape Crisis Centres

National network of women volunteers offering support, counselling, help as well as a safe place to women who have been raped or sexually assaulted. The national number can give details of local groups.

Write:
National Rape Crisis Centre, PO Box 69, London WC1X 9NJ
Phone:
071 837 1600 (24-hour crisis line)

Lesbian, Gay and Bisexual Organisations

London Lesbian and Gay Switchboard
24-hour advice/information daily on anything you can think of, including HIV.

Phone:
071 837 7324

London Lesbian Line
Information and advice on a range of matters for lesbians.

Phone:
071 251 6911 (Monday and Friday 2 p.m. to 10 p.m.; Tuesday to Thursday 7 p.m. to 10 p.m.)
  Both the above organisations should be able to give information about local groups/services.

Shakti – South Asian Lesbian and Gay Network

Write:
BM Box 3167, London WC1N 3XX
Phone:
071 837 2782 (daytimes – ask for Shakti)
081 993 9001 (evenings and weekends)

Drug Agencies

DAWN – Drugs, Alcohol, Women, Nationally
Advice, information and help to women with alcohol or other drug problems. Education and information, especially booklets.

Write:
Omnibus Workspace, 39 North Road, London N7 9DP

Phone:
071 700 4653

SCODA – Standing Conference on Drug Abuse
Coordinating body for non-statutory services and people working in the drugs field. Assists in development of services, training funding, runs conferences, produces leaflets and a guide to specialist drug services in England.

Write:
1–4 Hatton Place, Hatton Gardens, London EC1N 8ND

Phone:
071 831 3595

Scottish Drugs Forum
Coordinates drugs education and information in Scotland and has list of local drugs agencies in Scotland.

Write:
266 Clyde Street, Glasgow G1 4JH

Phone:
041 221 1175 (Monday to Friday 9.30 a.m. to 4.30 p.m.)

THE TERRENCE HIGGINS TRUST HIV/AIDS BOOK

Turning Point
National network of support centres for drug users and their friends and relatives.

Write:
9-12 Long Lane, London EC1A 9HA

Phone:
071 606 3947

People with Haemophilia

The Haemophilia Society
Advice and literature on living with haemophilia generally, as well as HIV-specific information.

Write:
123 Westminster Bridge Road, London SE1 7HR

Phone:
071 928 2020

The MacFarlane Trust
Charitable trust independent of the Haemophilia Society. Its only function is to distribute money from the government to people with HIV and AIDS.

Write:
PO Box 627, London SW1 0QG
Phone:
071 233 0342 (Monday to Friday, 2 p.m. to 5 p.m.)

INDEX

INDEX